Semiotic Perspectives on Clinical Theory and Practice

Approaches to Semiotics
98

Mouton de Gruyter
Berlin · New York

Semiotic Perspectives on Clinical Theory and Practice

Medicine, Neuropsychiatry and Psychoanalysis

Edited by

Bonnie E. Litowitz
Phillip S. Epstein

Mouton de Gruyter
Berlin · New York 1991

Mouton de Gruyter (formerly Mouton, The Hague)
is a Division of Walter de Gruyter & Co., Berlin.

⊗ Printed on acid-free paper which falls within the guidelines of the ANSI to ensure permanence and durability.

Library of Congress Cataloging in Publication Data

Semiotic perspectives on clinical theory and practice : medicine, neuropsychiatry, and psychoanalysis / edited by Bonnie E. Litowitz, Phillip S. Epstein.
p. cm. – (Approaches to semiotics ; 98)
Based partly on a conference held on March 14, 1987 at Rush-Presbyterian-St. Luke's Medical Center in Chicago.
Includes bibliographical references.
Includes index.
ISBN 0-89925-740-2 (cloth : alk. paper)
1. Psychoanalysis – Congresses. 2. Neuropsychiatry – Congresses. 3. Semiotic – Congresses. I. Litowitz, Bonnie E. II. Epstein, Phillip S., 1937– . III. Series.
[DNLM: 1. Communication. 2. Psychoanalysis. 3. Psychoanalytic Theory. 4. Symbolism (Psychology) W1 AP535 v. 98 / / WM 460 S471]
RC506.S46 1991
616.89'17 – dc20 91-7585
CIP

Die Deutsche Bibliothek – Cataloging-in-Publication Data

Semiotic perspectives on clinical theory and practice :
medicine, neuropsychiatry, and psychoanalysis / ed. by Bonnie E. Litowitz ; Phillip S. Epstein. – Berlin ; New York : Mouton de Gruyter, 1991
(Approaches to semiotics ; 98)
ISBN 3-11-012632-X
NE: Litowitz, Bonnie E. [Hrsg.]; GT

Printing: Werner Hildebrand, Berlin. – Binding: Lüderitz & Bauer, Berlin.
Printed in Germany.

Preface

On March 14, 1987, a conference on semiotics, psychiatry and psychoanalysis was held at Rush-Presbyterian-St. Luke's Medical Center in Chicago as part of the medical center's sesquicentennial celebration. Sponsored by the department of psychiatry, the goal was to introduce mental health professionals and academicians interested in psychoanalysis to semiotics as a new perspective on their work, whether clinical or theoretical. Many participants were exposed to semiotics for the first time; others were familiar with general semiotics but not with its application to clinical data and theory. Limitations of time and money impelled a focus on psychoanalytic theory that was narrower than desired, as one would have preferred to set that discussion within the broader context of related medical fields. This volume affords an opportunity to do just that.

The conference presentations form a nucleus which has been expanded to include solicited manuscripts on closely related topics: psychosomatic medicine; neuro-psychiatry; and pharmaco-biology. The connections between psychoanalysis, on the one hand, and these related fields, on the other, are both historical and contemporary. Freud was trained as a neurologist whose early work under the influence of Charcot and in collaboration with Breuer dealt directly with psychosomatic and neuropsychiatric disorders such as the conversion hysterias, obsessive-compulsive disorders, neurasthenias, and paranoias. And, he was a major contributor to the literature on the anesthetic properties of cocaine. Only gradually and reluctantly did he move from physical to purely psychological explanations in his symptomatology, always hoping that a truly "scientific" psychology would provide a basis in the brain for his theory of the mind; a theme Michael F. Basch will take up in this volume.

From the beginning, however, his theory was semiotic, invoking representations and memory traces. Distinguishing features of psychoanalytic (as opposed to, say, behavioral) psychology are its insistence on symptoms as symbolic representations and on the interpretation of meanings as foundational to curative change. In this regard, one could say that Lacan's dramatic rereading of Freud has revealed only what was already there, merely appearing exotic when viewed through the prism of French structural linguistics.

Recent advances in pharmacotherapies have radically altered both diagnosis and treatment of patients suffering from mental illnesses. Many of the types of patients whom Freud once saw in clinics for nervous and mental disorders are now advised to seek combinations of specific pharmacological and psychotherapeutic interventions. As the interface between neurobiology and psychology becomes more explicit, many theoreticians are hopeful that the hour of Freud's scientific psychology may be at hand.

It is fitting then that psychoanalysis serve as a gateway to what we hope will be renewed discussion of clinical and theoretical psychology, with semiotics providing a common perspective that can bridge the biological and the psychological. Interventions by hand (e.g., psychotropic drugs) and by word (e.g., therapeutic interpretations) are addressed by Eugen Baer and by Thure von Uexküll. Taking the perspective of Piaget's genetic epistemology, von Uexküll shows how the history of the discipline of medicine recapitulates individual ontogenesis: knowledge is created by each child first through hand-action and then through word-meanings. He argues for a synthesis of the two approaches, rather than a displacement of one by the other, especially in cases of psychosomatic illness. One finds here echoes of Niels Bohr's complementarity principle: not either-or but both-and: *Nur die Fülle führt zur Klarheit* ('Only wholeness leads to clarity').

Wholeness is addressed by Baer as he invokes a Platonic dialogue centering on the healing powers of *logoi kaloi*, beautiful words. He calls up the story of medicine, moving through three critical moments in its (his)story: knowledge and intervention that in the oracular period came from the Gods were given to expert men by Hippocrates, and finally to each individual by Freud. These transitions mark a shift in focus from soma to psyche and in curative power from other to self. After Freud, we find that the curative dialogue is not mediated by priests or doctors. The dialogue is within each individual and the story of medicine then becomes each person's (his)story. The psychoanalyst, like the philosopher, encourages the telling of that story in words that heal. The themes of these stories – life, death, health – are woven into different narratives by divided or split subjects, at once the teller and the told, in the eternal pursuit of meaning.

Both Arnold Goldberg and Barnaby B. Barratt take up the topics of narration and meaning. Goldberg describes current explanatory theories in the discipline of psychoanalysis as competing narratives. When psychoanalysis gives up its infantile (i.e., from its childhood) wish to have a scientific foundation embedded in neurology and brain, it is left with not one consensual foundation but with several alternate foundations; each one, a different story. Thus, hermeneutic sciences are destined to engage in the same eternal pursuit of meaning as the individual.

The pursuit of unconscious meaning, the *sine qua non* of any psychoanalytic treatment, is the topic of Barratt's paper. Barratt uses the pivotal psychoanalytic concept of the unconscious to radicalize the "semiotic revolution", one manifestation of our century's emphasis on language. While allowing that psychoanalysis is indeed a semiotic science, he argues for psychoanalysis' unique contribution by engaging three major figures from current interpretive debates: Lacan; Derrida;

and Kristeva. Again, the question of self and its other arises, with Barratt arguing for "nonidentity" and "contradictoriness".

Post-structuralist theoreticians note the death of the Cartesian subject and call into doubt the certitude of thinking and even of skepticism: you think you know your language, your history, your self, your thoughts or even what it means to know something – but you don't. However, even within this linguistic/semiotic revolution, Barratt argues, psychoanalysis forces a still more radical view of what it means to know something. He concludes with a description of Freudian knowledge as "anti-semiotic". Finally, since discovery and knowledge are the bases for science, Freud's radical science of the individual causes perturbations throughout every science by challenging the surety of knowledge and the unity of the knowing subject.

Without a fixed point of meaning need one despair; or, to paraphrase Italo Svevo (*The confessions of Zeno.* [trans. Beryl de Zoete.] New York: Vintage, 1958 [1923]), need one get seasick even if the world does go round? Baer concludes his retelling of medicine's story with "guidelines for praxis", three suggestions arising out of a semiotic perspective. One of these is to open up discussions of the belief systems of both doctors and their patients. Goldberg's variations on a theme of psychoanalysts at a case seminar and Barrett's exploration of psychoanalytic dialogue are two examples of the rich promise of this approach. They conclude not with despair but with a sense of liberation for a new perspective on science.

Nor should a semiotic perspective on science be confined to the hermeneutic and to mind as distinct from the biological and brain. F. Eugene Yates clearly illustrates the explanatory power of semiotic concepts in discussions of molecular systems. Even, and especially, at the biological level one cannot separate organism from environment, meaning from context. In pharmacological interventions one cannot separate drug chemistry from state of receptor sites. Effects can only be understood in terms of communicational exchanges and messages, codes and constraints. Yates argues that the realization that "steadiness is death" need not leave one unsteady. Although the easy path of reductionism is no longer viable, one need not therefore become lost among an infinite number of alternatives.

The topic of science and its genealogy runs through all these papers. The twentieth century has removed our constants (e.g., time), undermined our belief in objectivity (e.g., Heisenberg's uncertainty principle) and in foolproof proofs (e.g., Gödel), and left us with the cold comfort that everything is relative, that everything depends (literally, hangs from something else). But like Pablo Neruda's description (*Memorias: confiesco que he vivido.* Buenos Aires: Losada, 1974) of the raiding conquistadores who dropped the rounded vowels of Spanish out of their sacks of plundered gold, we are left with language as our new object/subject. In reviewing the fallout at mid-century of earlier explosions in quantum physics, Michael Riordan remarks:

> In retracing the steps taken in particle physics during the sixties and seventies, what impressed me most was the role of language in creating this reality ... This key role of language in creating physical reality gives an important hint about the nature of objectivity ... Those ideas that capture the allegiance of a scientific community become – at least for a time – the objective reality of that field. This objectivity is not 'the way things are', but the way they are understood and discussed by the great majority of its practitioners (*The hunting of the quark*. New York: Simon & Schuster, 1987: 368–9).

Thus, it was no coincidence that as science was spinning out quanta and quarks philosophy was taking a linguistic turn, a turn set in motion or at least presaged by Peirce's similar observation over one hundred years before: "The very origin of the conception of reality shows that this conception essentially involves the notion of community ... so that reality depends on the ultimate decision of the community" (*Philosophical writings of Peirce*. [Justus Buchler ed.] New York: Dover Publications,1955: 247 & 250).

Freud's new psychology both anticipated and propelled the hegemony of linguistic models. Bonnie E. Litowitz's paper rearticulates Freud's notions that we are constituted by language, as are our psychopathologies and their cure. Freud christened his new form of therapy the "talking cure"; but his insistence on using normal functioning (e.g., dreams, slips of the tongue, jokes) to demonstrate his new psychology is ample proof that his goal was not just a theory of deviation or disease, but a total theory of the mind. Litowitz argues that his use of the limiting metaphors of language (e.g., translations) and his abundant verbal examples obscure the clearly semiotic nature of his theory.

Throughout its history, psychoanalysis has maintained Freud's desire to make psychoanalysis a scientific psychology; taking one form in an ongoing debate about whether psychoanalysis is a science; and if so, what kind. Armed with Peirce's concept of abduction, Matthias Kettner enters that debate by challenging Grünbaum's recent criticism of psychoanalysis. Kettner argues that Peirce's innovative logical alternative to hypothetico-deductive reasoning has been underappreciated, demonstrating how abduction (in a form more expanded than originally proposed by Peirce) might clarify psychoanalytic epistemology. Here, then, is a third approach to psychoanalysis from a semiotic perspective, not as a theory of representation or as anti-semiotic, but as embodying a novel type of inference. Since abduction comes from within semiotic theory, Kettner's paper offers an alternate perspective on Barratt's claim that identifies semiotics necessarily with the "analytico-referential episteme". The idea that semiotic theory could make scientific reasoning clearer, and thus more fallible, was an original impetus for Peirce's pioneering work, and illustrates the further contribution of a semiotic perspective, beyond issues of representation and language.

Not everyone is equally willing to abandon Freud's quest for a scientific psychology founded in neurobiology and the brain to embrace a hermeneutic or semiotic approach. In his brief discussion of Barratt's paper, Basch argues for psycho-analysis' biological foundations, which he substantiates with a review of Freud's shifting positions on this issue. One finds here a reprise within the lengthy debate on psychoanalysis' status as a science of a theme Yates articulates at the molecular level. Both Basch and Yates are proponents of a unified theory of science in terms of informational exchanges at multiple levels; leading Basch to conclude that "psychology is an aspect of biology."

Semiotics as a means of unifying and classifying the sciences has a venerable history in the discipline (viz. Morris and Peirce). This self-conscious or reflexive use of a theory of signs to explain other sign phenomena is yet another promise of a semiotic perspective; namely, that we can span disparate historical moments in a discipline's history (e.g., medicine and psychoanalysis) or synthesize separate synchronic moments (e.g., biological and psychological functioning within one organism). For the science of signs, the different materialities of signs – chemical, biological, physical, imagic, verbal – pose no obstacle but become rather part of the inquiry. For the most part, however, it is language that receives the lion's share of attention.

A reexamination of the role of language in psychopathology underpins both Bernard Rubin's and Phillip S. Epstein's papers. Lacan's rereading of Freudian texts forms the foundation for Rubin's reevaluation of a clinical case of psychosis. The case materials from treatment records and a journal illustrate several Lacanian concepts: the privileging of the signifier over the signified (from French semiology); the constant gliding or movement of signifiers, exemplifying primary process displacements; a "lack" as organizing principle that drives the developmental progression from imaginary to symbolic registers, resulting in subjectivity and gender identification. Lacan's theory of psychosis depends upon a derailing of normal development prior to the child's entrance into the symbolic register or order. One consequence is the paranoid's "I", which is imaginary (although seemingly symbolic) and the eruption of symptoms in the "real" order (e.g., hallucinations, psychosomatic disorders). The case materials offer us a glimpse of the patient's (her)story, and provide specific instantiations of the themes from Baer's (his)story: life, death, health.

Another kind of lack or absence characterizes alexithymia, literally 'without words for moods'. Epstein's paper defines and gives the history of this symbolic disorder that has become a research focus in neuropsychiatry. Predating this recent label, however, are clinical descriptions of patients who tend to express their feelings through signs in the body (e.g., psychosomatic disorders) and who do not engage in the talking cure. Whether described as an emergence in the real and a foreclosure from the symbolic or as somatoform disorders and psychoses, Epstein argues that a reinterpretation of psychiatric categories from a semiotic perspective holds the promise of new insights. For, the reading of symptoms as/and signs is the basis of medical semiotics as well as the earliest roots of semiotics in medicine.

Wittgenstein's proclamation heralded the opening of the twentieth century: the limits of my language are the limits of my world. Much of the intellectual history of the ensuing years has been a working out of that programme – two kinds of structural linguistics (descriptive and not); natural language processing and artificial intelligence; the philosophy of language (versus linguistic philosophy) and speech act theory; information theory and cybernetics; transformational and post-transformational grammars; critical literary theory and narratology; semiology and semiotics – to name but a few. We are now at the end of the century still not sure where our boundaries and limits are, if we are on or over the edge. A major force in the intellectual history of this century has been psychoanalysis, which refuses to accept as final Wittgenstein's comment; namely, what we cannot speak about we must pass over in silence. In this context, the value of the present volume is that it both reflects these same concerns and contributes to the discourse about them, which is, after all, but another episode in our-story.

These, then, are the themes of the papers in this volume: scientific paradigms and the problems of knowledge; the refracted subject of knowing – divided, real, imagined, symbolic; and the sign systems at all levels that constitute, express and ultimately subvert both science and subjectivity. These themes are not taken up in turn so much as interwoven throughout, within and between these papers. The order of presentation of the papers reflects a disciplinary focus, from general to particular: from medicine and physiology to neuropsychiatry, psychoanalysis, and Lacanian psychoanalysis. The following authors presented some version of their papers at the 1987 conference: Eugen Baer, Barnaby B. Barratt, Michael F. Basch, Arnold Goldberg, Bonnie E. Litowitz, and Bernard Rubin. (Françoise Meltzer also presented at the conference but was unable to participate in this volume.) Phillip S. Epstein, Matthias Kettner, Thure von Uexküll, F. Eugene Yates contributed the additional articles from related fields.

We are deeply grateful to all the authors for their willing participation in this publication. From the beginning Jan Fawcett, chairman of the psychiatry department at Rush-Presbyterian-St.Luke's Medical Center, the department faculty as a whole, and especially Robert Zadylak provided the enthusiastic support that made the conference and this subsequent publication possible. We are thankful that the

Sesquicentennial Committee considered this topic a fitting salute for the institution's 150th birthday and provided necessary funding. The generosity of the George B. and Mary A. Young Fund for Scholars in Health Education, Research, Policy and in Psychiatry and the Humanities is especially appreciated. Finally, we extend heartfelt thanks to Alan Lipton for his skillful assistance in preparing the manuscripts and to the Humanitas Institute for their support services. We reserve a special note of appreciation for Thomas A. Sebeok who mentored and midwifed this project in his inimical manner; guiding, advising, assisting, enabling and all the other gerunds that it takes to make things happen. He is the master jack-of-all-trades in semiotics and he put each to use for us.

Contents

Note on citations

Citations of Freud in the text refer to the *Standard Edition of the complete psychological works of Sigmund Freud* (S.E.), translated from the German under the general editorship of James Strachey, in collaboration with Anna Freud, assisted by Alix Strachey and Alan Tyson, published in London by The Hogarth Press (1953-1974). Similarly, G.W. refers to the *Gesammelte Werke*, under the editorship of Anna Freud et al., published in London by the Imago Publishing Co. (1940-1952). Numerals following S.E. or G.W. refer to the volume(s) and page(s) of cited materials.

Throughout this volume, for references with two dates, the first is the date of original publication and the second, that of the edition used by the author.

Semiotic presuppositions of healing: the story of medicine

Eugen Baer

A good story attracts
but does not explain.

Introduction

I would like first to explain the title. The phrase, the story of medicine, can mean at least two things. *As genitivus obiectivus* it means the story one can tell about medicine, hence a kind of historiography, a history of medicine. As *genitivus subjectivus* it suggests that medicine is itself a story in the sense that it can be seen as a narrative in which actors (physicians, patients) work together toward some goal of transformation, for instance to restore health or to prolong life. Here medicine is seen as a form of literature, specifically as a form of self-representation or autobiography.

The term, autobiography, shows that the two senses are interrelated in that we have in both cases descriptions of identity (answering the question: what is healing?), one stretched out over time, historical, the other more structural and paradigmatic. I am going to speak about both senses of medical stories. Moreover, I will be practicing philosophy, that is, I will be interested in conceptual presuppositions that can be discovered in any description of healing. I call these presuppositions semiotic because they involve processes with which therapists are very familiar, namely inferences, and inferences are based on signs.

First, then, a glimpse at a semiotic history of medicine. Later, in a second part, a short survey of medicine as a form of implied literary self-presentation. Both parts revolve around four fundamental concepts of healing: *health, disease, life and death.* A third and final part will provide a few guidelines for praxis.

1. Historical sketch of medical semiotics

The question where to begin is important for semiotics, because beginnings, properly speaking, are impossible once one enters the sign. The very notion of beginning conceptually implies a state before the beginning. Every beginning is thus a sign of a state preceding it which undermines the very notion of a beginning. For example, I may say that our conference[1] begins today, but by saying it, I posit a space before this conference which integrally belongs to it, were it only by way of preparing this talk and planning to come. Signs posit a difference, for example *before/after*, but they erase that difference at the same time. They have it both ways, and these two ways (of having the cake and eating it too) will occupy us here, because they represent two states of consciousness, one formless, the other formed, which are at the same time one consciousness. So where do I begin my historical sketch of medicine? I will begin with Plato.

1.1. The lost object of medicine

Whitehead (1967) once superbly described Plato's place in philosophy by saying that Western intellectual history was a series of footnotes to his work. I subscribe to this but with a twist insofar as Plato who marks the beginning of medical semiotics is already a latecomer and forever belated, precisely because he marks a beginning. The work I am alluding to is entitled *Charmides*. It is one of Plato's earlier dialogues (1961) which are notorious for all ending in Socratic *aporia*, a complete loss of way and orientation, so that the end of the dialogue is really its beginning but in such a way that by now it has become clear that everything is always just beginning.

The dialogue begins with an encounter of Socrates and Charmides. Charmides is at that time (around 432 B.C.) the talk of the town, a youth whose beauty represents the Greek ideal of a sound body. There is just some minor irritating thing about him: sometimes, when he wakes up in the morning, he has a headache. On the pretense that Socrates is a doctor who can heal his headache, Charmides is introduced to Socrates, and now something startling happens. Socrates, completely baffled by the beauty of the youth, is for a moment speechless and quite besides himself. We have here probably the only place in Plato's entire work where Socrates loses control of himself. The absence of the word (*logos*) in the presence of such a beautiful body (*soma*) is significant not only to set up the typically Greek contrast between *soma* and *psyche*, but also to show the power of the body to absorb the mind and to declare itself the sole reality. This is indeed, as Socrates sees it, the fate of Greek medicine: it is in love with the body only. For a brief moment, we see Socrates act out the fate of a medicine which has lost its speech. As he comes to and finds his words again, he tells the story of an older and strange medicine, one which is in love with words. "When I was serving in the army up north," he tells Charmides, "I met one of those Thracian doctors of Zalmoxis, the local king and god of the dead. These doctors are said to make men immortal. He told me that most diseases elude the Greek doctors because they have the wrong notion of wholeness. The body is only a part of a larger whole, the soul (*psyche*), which is the source both of bodily health and bodily disease. And if the Greek doctors do not pay any attention to the soul, they miss the whole boat, because if the whole (soul) is not in good condition, it is impossible that the part (body) should be" (Plato 1961: 103).

Socrates is launching here an attack on Hippocratic medicine (1923), coupled with an attempt to reintroduce an element it has lost, namely the soul. The soul has to be cured first if the body is to be healthy. And the soul is cured by certain charms which consist of 'beautiful words' (*logoi kaloi*). As a result of these words, the soul begins to think in a healthy way and once the soul does that, physical ailments are seen in their proper place and can be treated with drugs.

So far as the story goes, it is surprisingly modern after 2500 years. The question is, what is this lost object of medicine? What is the meaning of *psyche*, and just how is *psyche* going to be the source of bodily health? Is it some kind of mind over matter, something that could shed light on the nature of psychosomatic disease?

Let us begin with the first question. What does the word *psyche* refer to? An apparently simple answer is to say that *psyche* refers to that in us which says "I". Whatever this word refers to, it seems to be the lost object of medicine that Plato mourns. Who is this "I"? It is, in each case, the speaking person. What is a speaking person? Who is it that speaks? Who am I as a speaker? The ancient and strange medicine which Plato evokes in *Charmides* seems to address this question as the key to a cure which is so radical that it is said to make men immortal.

1.2. Self-knowledge and medicine

But now we ask, what does self-knowledge, also called *sophia* (wisdom), have to do with medicine? Socrates says that *sophia* is generated in the *psyche* by beautiful words which charm the dead and make humans immortal. As Socrates administers the charm, it becomes clear that the Socratic dialogue itself is the charm. What is going on in this dialogue? How does it charm the dead, and just how can it grant immortality? And what happens to Charmides' headache? In approaching these questions, we sketch a mini-treatise of medical semiotics.

First, what is going on in the dialogue? Socrates wants to find out whether Charmides is already thinking in a healthy way so that he can give him the pretended drug for his headache. So the two go searching for a tenable definition of *sophrosyne*, mostly translated as 'temperance' but in fact synonymous with *sophia* or self-knowledge. The dialogue goes from definition to definition, each one breaking down and forcing the two speakers to start again. The dialogue ends in *aporia*, a loss of way. There are seemingly no positive, only negative results. In this sense, the dialogue is a failure. It does not tell us what *psyche* is. It leaves us entirely in the dark. But maybe it is precisely this darkness that gives us a clue to the grammar of the word "I". It may just be the case that *aporia* is an integral element of self-knowledge, that an important part of the grammar of the word "I" has to do with a complete loss of way, with the darkness of the mind.

1.3. Medicine and ignorance

Let us suppose that this is indeed the case. We would then have a rather startling insight into Socrates' notion of the role of ignorance in medicine. A medicine which includes the speaking person and begins the art of healing with an investigation of the word, is framed and suspended by the knowledge of ignorance, by an ability to sustain a state of ongoing transition from knowledge to ignorance, an ability to follow one's mind into the darkness of not knowing: *oida ouden eidenai*, 'I know that I know nothing'. The knowledge that we know nothing is indeed so strange that we might be tempted to dismiss its relevance for medicine altogether, since nothing is not something that is likely to make a contribution to anything, let alone to such a complicated matter as medicine.

The statement, I know that I know nothing, says in one reading that I know my own knowing as being not so, that my knowledge is pretended knowledge, that I do not know at all. In another reading, the statement says that the true object of my knowledge sooner or later stares nothingness in the eye, stands eye to eye with itself and sees nothing at all. In each case we have a kind of mirror-relation of knowledge with itself and by implication of the "I" with itself. It seems that when the "I" sees itself, it sees nothing at all or, rather, that whatever appears in the mirror as a figure of the "I" is really nothing.

1.4. The dia-logic of the self

Plato introduces here into Western philosophy a dia-logic of the self which practices a division of the speaking subject into knowing and known which at the same time is a paradoxical division of a subject whose knowing is not knowing. We can notice similar movements toward the same division much earlier in the Vedas of India and later in Buddhism (Griffiths 1986, Hume 1971). Both movements created very far reaching practices of healing whose histories are an integral part of any history of medicine (Baer 1988, 1989).

I reserve an analysis of this division of subjectivity for later. For now I concentrate on the experience it produces in Socratic dialogue. It is this experience which is crucial for medical semiotics and which says, in effect, that my story is impossible.

1.5. The impossible story

What do I mean by story here? I mean autobiography. I mean those words which would say the truth about me. The story is the word about my self that would give it meaning. Socratic questioning attempts to formulate such a story. For example, it attempts to find the meaning of the word "I". It does not find it or, rather, any finding turns out to be inadequate. The story which I tell about myself, my autobiography, seems to be impossible. We will come back to that.

It is this impossibility of our story which is assumed in Socratic dialogue as being a part of the cure. But by doing that Socrates leaves you and me in the dark. It is the darkness of stepping beyond, the darkness of the abyss, the darkness of an interdict. And it is precisely this darkness that Hippocrates took off the shoulders of medicine in a moment of medical history and whose impact on the subsequent course of medicine cannot be overestimated.

1.6. The Hippocratic moment

Plato gives us a clue for seeing the Hippocratic moment as a constitutive moment of repression in medical history which, like many repressions, makes possible a certain success. The major accomplishment of Hippocrates consists in moving the medical field from the divine to the secular. He eliminates a specifically divine causality for diseases like epilepsy and impotence. He pulls medicine out of the dark age of Apollo's oracle at the temple of Delphi and leaves to the oracle only medicine's "leftover", that for which medicine has as yet no cure.

Plato intervenes here with a double gesture: on the one hand he continues Hippocrates' move from the divine to the secular, on the other he reverses it by adding *logos* to *physis*, the laws of the word to the laws of nature. We can look at this also as a series of shifts of the field of medicine: Hippocrates shifts medicine from the divine to nature; Plato adds yet another shift from nature to the word. For Socrates, the medical field is constituted not only *physei*, by the laws of nature, it is constituted in a much larger sense *nomo*, by the laws of the word (cf. *Phaedrus*).

We may ask: what is it that the word adds to medical practice? For Plato, its contribution is not to be despised. The word adds meaning to the whole thing. It addresses questions such as: what are we doing when we pursue well-being, in the first place? What is health? What disease? When can I consider myself to be cured? And so on.

1.7. A mini-history of medicine

As soon as the meaning-question is raised in medicine, the history of medicine appears in a new light. I detect in it three moments which are all contained in the moment of the Socratic *eros*. The first moment is the moment of the oracle, spanning back to the third millenium B.C. which, side by side with surgical and herbal medicine, saw in the oracular word a healing connection between the present and the future, the living and the dead, mortals and immortals. The second moment is the moment of Hippocrates who, by excluding the oracular word, constitutes medicine as an investigation into the natural causes of health and disease. The third moment is the moment of Freud who (re)discovers the role of the oracular word in its role of "speaking cure".

The three moments are contained in Plato's notion of the medical process as dialogue. Plato affirms the biological level of medicine but finds it incomplete without the question of meaning, supplied by the word, which provides the scene in which the story of medicine can unfold. This scene is language.

Once language becomes the object of medical discourse, once the subject, symbolized by the word "I", attempts to speak the truth about itself, we enter an infinite regression (or progression) of meaning. The accent is here on infinite. Socratic dialogue assists in the birth of meaning whose completion is infinitely delayed. It seems that the incompleteness of meaning is part of meaning itself. Meaning therefore cannot be itself. It is always just about to be or has just ceased to be. The word stands in the middle between this "not yet" and "already too old". Its fragile ontology consists in bridging that which as yet has no being with that whose being has just expired. In the middle we find the impossibility of being, the impossibility of the present, of presence without absence, of life without death. Such is the dialogic, the twofold logic of the self. The major task, therefore, of Socratic autobiography is to affirm and assume one's own absence to one's own story. This is the true birth of the self, the scope of the Socratic maieutic.

1.8. The word as midwife

The Socratic word which assists in the birth of the divided self is a word which is presence and absence at once. It is a word which cuts the word "I" in two dimensions and induces in it a division whose oneness cannot be represented.

This division is a product of language, an effect of its peculiar grammar which insists that subjectivity can represent itself only by accepting its own absence to the presence it constructs for itself. In other words, when we try to answer the question, who is it that is having an illness?, the subject of illness, the patient, disappears. And medicine finds itself suddenly without a subject.

The word brings forth the presence of the "I" as an absence, as a "not-I". My own absence to myself, which I can only formulate as a negation or absence of my "I", is a part of myself. So here we have this strange logical conclusion of medical semiotics again: that in order to be me I have not to be me. I exist, so to speak, on the stages of two different theaters simultaneously, one in which I function as I, another, in which there is not an I. This other scene (*der andere Schauplatz*), the one in which I am not an I, must be logically postulated from the grammar of words, but it cannot be represented. It has to remain unconscious. This was Freud's great (re)discovery. About 2500 years after the oracular word was eliminated from medicine by Hippocrates, Freud tried to reintroduce it by discovering the grammar of dream words.

1.9. The antithetical grammar of words

In an article published in 1910 and entitled "The antithetical meaning of primal words", Freud thought he had found in the work of the linguist Abel a confirmation for this claim that in the unconscious a word like *good* could also mean *bad*, *far* could mean *near*, in short, dream words meant not only themselves but their opposites too. Abel believed he had found in Ancient Egyptian an insinuation for such an antithetical use of words, and although his thesis has been disconfirmed by Egyptologists on historical grounds, I believe that his and Freud's thesis is absolutely correct on semantic grounds. From a semiotic perspective, to say a word I need to say its opposite too, because a meaning arises only in some kind of contrast to another meaning. For example, the word "I" has no meaning in itself. It needs to enter a contrast to acquire meaning, and the widest possible contrast is achieved by negation, represented by the contradictory "not-I". The notion of an "I" includes therefore that of a "not-I" as belonging to its identity, while at the same time it has to exclude it as not belonging to it. Identity has its root in a contradiction and can therefore not be represented. It is semantically empty or all-inclusive. It does not mean a thing. Only by suppressing its contradictory part can identity appear, but it will always appear as something which is in search of its contradictory (cf. Plato's *Symposium*). Only by suppressing the not-I can the ego appear as a fragment of the I. The speaking subject arises from a repression which is semiotically absolutely necessary.

Medical semiotics sees therefore the Freudian unconscious as a necessary repression of a contradictory signifier (Freud 1925). The repression is necessary because the meanings of words coarise with their opposites and these opposites cannot be simultaneously affirmed without doing away with meaning. The contradiction, for example, of being simultaneously ego and alter, mortal and immortal, alive and dead, marks therefore the impossible place of desire (*eros*), from where all speaking proceeds and toward which it tends. Our stories are all spoken from a place of impossibility.

1.10. The impossible story revisited

Freud saw in the antithetical meaning of words the regressive and archaic character of the expression of dream thoughts. He saw the same mechanism at work in those errors of speech in which we say the opposite of what we consciously intend to say. For the semiotician, the contradictory semantic field of any word is a logical necessity. If there is anything archaic or regressive in this, it is so in the sense of finding the *arche*, the origin, of meaning, and finding it in a contraction.

Freud thought of himself as a translator of the archaic space of the dream into the civilized space of the ego. *Wo Es war soll Ich werden* translates literally into 'where It was I shall come to be' rather than the accepted 'where id was, there ego shall be' (Freud 1933). Freud (re)discovered in the place of the transpersonal "It" the other scene of speaking, this other theater, in which words mean also their opposites and in comparison to which the conscious "I" does not really know what it is saying. He knew further that this other scene was the *arche*, the origin, of the meaning of the patient's life, and that an analysis of this impossible origin was interminable. Psychoanalysis was mostly helping patients to acquire a kind of knowledge which would allow them to know that they did not know.

I would say that the knowledge about this other place, like the knowledge about the blind spot in dreams which he could not analyse, was the knowledge about a notion of health which is not only archaic but truly prehistorical and even preontological in the sense that this semantically blind spot does not enter the patient's history at all, while at the same time holding it in trans-semantic and therefore transtemporal suspense. It is from this blind spot that our life story proceeds toward that kind of successful failure which Freud (1933) called *Fehlleistung*, 'parapraxis'. It is a failure, because the analysand's story cannot reveal his/her identity except as some kind of (hopefully) liberating illusion; "successful", because beyond all identity, the analysand's discourse proceeds from a space which remains semantically empty and open and as such rejoins the erotic openness of the Socratic dialogue.

1.11. Four fundamental concepts of medicine

With Freud's rediscovery of the speaking cure, my mini-history of medical semiotics rejoins its oracular beginnings where the word was the largest possible framework for medicine. The word was internal, not external, to healing. With words, we not only speak about our life, about health and disease. Rather, the notions of health and disease are effects or products of the way we speak them. Language is not only about medicine; it is medicine itself in the sense that it provides medicine with its basic concepts without which the practice of medicine becomes meaningless. Such concepts are: health, disease, death, and life.

I am going to provide a systematic semiotic analysis of these four concepts in a moment. But let me very briefly summarize the results of our mini-history in terms of these four notions. Health refers to a state in which we assume the infinite openness of our story as a part of ourselves. A part of us is necessarily blind. It is by assuming this blindness that we achieve, like the blind seers of ancient times, the deepest vision of our life as a story which proceeds from a space of impossibility. Medical semiotics has therefore a double charge vis-à-vis medicine: (1) to show patients that it is normal if their life stories do not make sense; and (2) to speak with patients about the impossibility of speaking.

Conversely, disease is then seen as a state of fixed and therefore false beliefs, of actions which proceed from such false beliefs. Here the contribution of medical semiotics might be to show that beliefs are necessary but impossible, and that all healing should be accompanied by strategies to free patients from attachments to beliefs.

Death, thirdly, is a state in which apparently all mental and physical activities are extinct. This corresponds to that aspect of our being in which meaning collapses. The task for medical semiotics here might be to facilitate access of patients toward this other side of us where the notion of "I" does not make sense. It is our preontological side which Buddhist medicine has practiced for millenia.

Finally, life is seen as an ongoing coming to birth in the word whose antithetical horizon invites us at all times to celebrate nirvana in the many physical and mental forms that come our way. Medical semiotics could contribute to a medical picture in which disease reminds us of a life that proceeds from death. This would mean concretely to work out ways in which patients can participate in the transition from their own preontology to their being, from their own absolute prehistory to actually entering their particular histories in free and constructive ways.

2. Medicine as literature

We are now ready to move from telling stories or histories about medicine to viewing medicine itself as a kind of story. How can one view medicine as a story? Suppose you ask people involved in medical practice what it is they are doing. If they tell you what they are doing they give you a description of their activity. They might say, for example, "as a physician, I try to prolong people's lives, to cure their diseases, etc." Or they might say, as patients, "I have come here to get my annual check-up", or something to that effect. Whatever they are saying, they are, viewed in literary terms, dramatizing their actions.

We can thus see the transition from medicine to medicine-as-literature as a transition from medical action to the description of medical action. I suggest that in making this move we are opening up the entire field of medical semiotics. We are confronting medicine with the question of meaning ('What is it you are doing here?') and we are given a response in terms of dramatic action ("I cure diseases"). We are given a medical narrative, and medical semiotics explores the logical implications of such narratives.

A first thing we have to say about medical narratives is that they are always autobiographical narratives, insofar namely as factual statements imply the beliefs of those making these statements. These beliefs might be such that they do not withstand rational scrutiny, and if that is the case, then medicine itself could be sick in the sense of suffering from wrong beliefs. It is entirely possible that the field of medicine suffers from language, that is, from the way it frames its own story. Medical semiotics addresses this language and, if applicable, offers treatment. This brings the approach of medical semiotics into close proximity to psychoanalysis.

Asked about his real achievement in developing psychoanalysis, Freud once said that he had taken a field of medicine, psychiatry, and turned it over to literature. What medical semiotics tries to do, is to turn the entire field of medicine over to literature. The phrase, medicine and literature, takes on an entirely new meaning: medicine is seen as a kind of literature. And literature is, broadly speaking, concerned with the meaning or absence of meaning in our daily living and dying. The move from medicine to medical semiotics is the move from trying to save lives to trying to make sense of saving lives.

This all has basically to do with the notion of "story". When physicians and patients describe their medical experience, when they formulate it in words, when they render explicit what they do implicitly, they become characters in their own story. Stories carry with them certain logical implications without which a story would never arise but which do not as such appear in the story. They are, so to speak, "behind" the story and we have to infer them, using the story as a sign.

I am selecting two such implications which will serve as the basic framework for summarizing the scope of medical semiotics. The first implication is the subject-object structure of identity statements. Hegel (1967) saw in this structure the minimal condition of any philosophical statement. In narratology, it is usually presented as the distinction between narrator and narrative (Rosenstock-Huessy 1970).

2.1. The narrating I and the narrated I

Generally speaking, semiotics is haunted by the difference and identity of presence and absence, because this is one of the definitions of the sign. When it comes to the narrative of medicine itself – and we now understand by "medical narrative" the various dramatizations of healing – we have first of all to distinguish between a narrator and the narrative, between a narrating "I" and a narrated "I", and then we have to say that the "I" is marked by this doubleness of subject and object which it assumes in the act of speech.

So when medicine presents itself as a story in all those ways in which the medical staff and patients represent themselves, we have on the one hand the narrated autobiographies or fragments thereof, and on the other the narrators. And although these two are one in the act of narration, they are at the same time separated from each other by an infinite abyss. And in this abyss lies the most radical root of health and disease.

Why? Because the speaking subjectivity is both internal and yet radically external to that which it says about itself. It is a fatal mistake to identify what I say about myself with myself. The story I utter is existentially my story since it presupposes my uttering it. But in terms of meaning it can never be my story. And this is something we have to look into more closely.

2.2. Tautology and autobiography

Grammatically, the simplest identity statement is already a doubling: I am I. Informationally speaking, such a statement is redundant; it is a tautology. It does not give us any information. It is completely empty. At the same time we all know that, if everything is said and done, the statement, I am I, is the deepest and most informative thing you could ever say about yourself. So what is going on here? How does tautology relate to autobiography?

Tautology means etymologically 'speech about the self' or 'speech about the same'. Grammatically it means that the subject and the predicate are the same, the same self, that is: I am I. But while this is true in the sense of reference, it is false in terms of grammatical form. The first "I" is in the place of the subject. The second "I" is the objective case of the pronoun. This is sometimes expressed by the phrase: I am me. A transformation has occurred from subject to object within the same semantic space of the pronoun "I". Can we neglect it? Hardly. Because for any statement of identity, language forces me to use this transformation. It is as if, grammatically speaking, I could never say who I am.

Notice that I am not at all speaking about content here. I am just referring to the grammatical form of a tautology which reveals at least two things: (1) a subject can only appear as an object. Without becoming empirical in some objective way, the subject has no being and is in this sense preontological; (2) while appearing only in objective form, the subject nevertheless transcends radically all its forms, because the pronoun's objective case can never take the place of the grammatical subject. In this sense the subject, although it appears in objective form, nevertheless never really appears as a subject. Every objective case of the "I" is only a sign of the "I" and as such a presence of an absence. The objective formulation of the "I" signals the absence of the "I" as a subject. Autobiography is tautology. No objective form can capture the speaking subject. This is why the tautology, I am I, although the emptiest statement in terms of information theory, is the fullest thing I can say about myself in terms of semiotic theory, because by rendering present my aboriginal emptiness, I breach a way toward wholeness and, since health is derived from wholeness, I point toward a notion of health which includes my absence and therefore makes me full.

2.3. Health

Health would then refer to that state of my being in which I can affirm, besides my presence, also my absence, which is a radical absence because it is not just a matter of memory but of logic. It is not that I cannot fully retain who I am, it is that it is logically impossible to know who I am. Health, from a semiotic perspective, is the acceptance and the experience of this impossibility.

Let me unfold this paradox a little. Medicine takes place within a story which is concerned with prolonging our life and delaying our death. When we enter this story and participate in it by narrating our own story (autobiography), we soon realize that our story cannot be told. It is impossible to close a text for reasons which are internal to the text. One such reason is that the narrating "I" eclipses itself in the very act of narration. The narrating "I" takes on objective form when it speaks, but this form cannot be identified with the "I", because it is only a part of it. In order, therefore, to get to the "I", I have to leave all objective form. But when I do that, instead of getting to the "I", I get nowhere.

Now this sounds vaguely familiar, i.e., lose your self so that you may find it, but it is not for that reason more understandable. And yet it seems to be a grammatical imperative. How can we understand it? I believe that based on the logic of the narrating I, we have to conclude that part of our being is forever unconscious, beyond any possible consciousness. This part is present in our speech, but as an absence. It is present in our consciousness, but as the unconscious.

Is this not contradictory? How can I be aware of the unconscious? Only if consciousness is itself a sign. A sign of what? I will give a more systematic answer shortly when I talk about death. For now we can say that consciousness is a sign of its own absence. Accordingly, we can be aware of something beyond consciousness. It is, as Freud once noted, the awareness of an outside world (*Außenwelt*) which is not exterior to consciousness but interior. There is something in consciousness which is beyond consciousness. This something, which by definition cannot be a something, is subjectivity.

Where I am a subject, on this perpetually other scene, I cannot assume any predicate, although all predicates are predicates only because they constitute and are supported by a subject. To be more precise, the predicate of subjectivity is that of being beyond all predicates.

The oldest philosophy we know, the one which originated in the Vedas of ancient India, knew about this formlessness of subjectivity. They knew that to superimpose a predicate on the subject was the category mistake *par excellence.* For us latecomers it is not so easy to see health as that part of us which is hidden from us by the very act of narrating our story. The place from which we speak and into which we speak cannot be represented. Words that help us enter this space of impossibility are, as Plato puts it, 'beautiful words' (*logoi kaloi*), words which heal. Such words are Socratic words which give birth to *eros*. By contrast, words that close up that space of unrepresentability are words which spell disease.

2.4. Disease

Who is it that has a disease? Who is health? If the speaking subject is beyond predicates, can it be said to be anything, let alone healthy or diseased? Obviously not. Health is after all an objectification of the "I", a predicate. But what is claimed here is that this predicate, healthy, applies only if the speaking subject accepts its own absence from the predication. I am healthy when I realize that the statement, I am healthy (or diseased), cannot be identified with myself.

The other scene of speaking causes all my speech about myself and about the world to fail. Autobiography is necessarily post-lapsarian language, after the fall. My speech is an ongoing *lapsus linguae*. I now say, in whatever I say, either too little or too much, or really both, since they come to be the same thing. I say too little, because nothing I could say about myself holds any water. And I say too much because by actually employing categories like "I" and "not-I" in my description I misleadingly suggest some kind of entities which are bearers of attributes.

In the middle between too little and too much we have the truth defined as the *adequatio rei et intellectus*, the equation between the thing and the intellect or, slightly modified, between the real and language. But this equation is impossible. Language cannot say the real; language always lies when it says the truth, because it can only work through repression. I cannot say the truth about myself; because my subjectivity is lacking in everything I say about myself.

The tautology, I am I, therefore states the truth as a lie. It is full and empty, true and false, possible and impossible. This is the reason why I am and am not who I think I am. As we saw, health resides in this ability to accept both as integral parts of my story which thereby becomes at once necessary and impossible.

By contrast, disease can be defined as the madness which consists in believing that we are who we think we are. This can be disastrous, no matter whether we believe we are Napoleon or John Smith. By closing the gap between the narrating I and the narrated I, we are creating the illusion that it is actually the "I" which is looking at itself. However, when I look at myself, I am always other. What is more, the look with which I look at myself, is always the look of the other.

2.5. The look of the other

Very generally speaking, medical semiotics sees disease as a fixation of the "I". Such a fixation is facilitated by the subject-object structure of identity. Language seduces us to mis-take the objective case of the "I" for the subject. We forget that my being, insofar as it can be cognized, is always in quotation marks. Our autobiography is pure citation. To put it succinctly: we are a quote.

But the question is, from what text do we cite when we quote ourselves? The answer is simple: we always quote from other quotes. Any text is essentially a citation insofar as it is necessarily supported by a subject which, however, cannot enter its own citation without citing itself. So another way of defining disease from a semiotic point of view is to say that it consists in the elision of the quotation marks which surround autobiographical statements. We forget the speaker. We thereby destroy the text as text and make of it an object. Disease points in the direction of the objectification of the "I". Health points in the other direction, the de-objectification of the "I".

In a manner of speaking, this is a matter of looking. If we replace the terms, narrating I and narrated I, with the scopic metaphor, observing I and observed I, we can see that the "I" is constituted as an object by the "I" itself, and it is constituted as such grammatically as the objective case of the "I". Grammar requires that when the "I" is looking at itself, it is always looking at its other. The same grammar also wants it that when I look at my own looking I have to see it as the look of the other. Both my seeing as well as that which is seen are objective cases of the "I". The most radical root of disease lies in grammar.

The look, which is always the look of the other, turns me into a picture. The grammar of identity statements requires that the observing "I" exclude itself from its own self-portrait. When I say I am myself, I turn out to be the other. The tautology, I am I, is therefore equivalent to the statement, I am the other.

We can see now how the first implication of narratology which I characterized as the distinction between the narrating I and the narrated I harbors a second implication, equivalent to the first but wider in its semantic application. This is the notion that opposite terms, like "I" and "other", constitute each other and are thus jointly the same. Buddhists call this grammatical phenomenon "dependent co-origination".

2.6. Dependent co-origination

The idea is relatively simple, but to feel its impact seems to be less simple. Semiotically, one can learn to view words, signs, things, events, and the like, as being empty and meaningless, unless they are given meaning by some other word, sign, or thing. So you need at least two contrasting things to have one meaning. In sem-iotics, one is two. This sounds contradictory, and it is. The consequence is that one cannot be said; identity is impossible. The logic of identity fails on logical ground; it is a failed and failing logic, a mistake, a parapraxis.

When I say a word like *you*, the word assumes meaning only in a space which contains the contradictory signifier *not-you*. The word *you* therefore contains intrinsically its contradictory, *not-you.* This can be unfolded by distinguishing two logical steps: (1) a state in which you and not you are one; and (2) a state in which you and not-you are two. Semiotically, these two states must be taken together. I would say, they are one, but I cannot say that really, because by now all oneness is by definition, i.e. by the force of grammar, twoness. The result seems to be disastrous. We are faced with a semantics in which opposites (1) mean the same, and (2) are nevertheless and because of it, differentiated. Good and evil are the same, but different. You and I are the same, but different; mortals and immortals are the same, but different. How are we to understand such nonsense?

Hegel tried to develop a logic along these lines. At the beginning of his *Phenomenology* (1967), he gives us a humorous grammar of indexical words, such as *this, I, here, now.* He shows that these words which denote in each case the most concrete and unique circumstance, are at the same time the most abstract and general words. Here we have thus a case of *concrete* and *abstract, unique* and *general, full* and *empty, immediate* and *mediate*, being the same. Viewed as sheer indexicals, words like *this, I, here, now* mean all cases of *this, I*, etc. Whatever *this* happens to be is *this.* Whatever *I* happen to be, *I* am. Wherever I happen to be, is *here.* Whenever I am, I am *now.* We see from this logic that the indexical *I* means all 'I's', *here* means all 'here's', *this* means all 'this's', *now* means all 'now's'. But in a universe in which *now* means all 'now's', it is never now. The word has lost its meaning. It has died before our very eyes. And it has died, because we took it seriously as what it was, namely, a word. If this word happens to be the pronoun I, we can witness the meaningful death of the "I" and are then able to formulate a semiotic perspective of death.

2.7. Death

To recapitulate: Words are empty of meaning, unless I introduce an instance of otherness. But once otherness is introduced as part of a word's meaning, the word's meaning is gone. The very element which gives meaning, takes it away. An example: the pronoun I takes on meaning only in contrast to a not-I. But once not-I is part of the meaning of "I", "I" means both "I" and "not-I" and therefore means nothing. How is meaning possible, then? Only on the ground of some repression, as we shall see. But notice for now, how words very naturally dissolve themselves into nothing. The claim is that if we take words seriously, we can witness their instantaneous death and thereby gain access to a semiotic formulation of what Buddhists call *nirvana* (Grimstone 1977).

This mysterious death of words which coexists with their lives applies to all words, including the word *Being.* If *being* contains, as part of its meaning, 'nothingness', then I am moved not only beyond language, but beyond the word *beyond.* Why is that so?

2.8. The dance of Shiva

Let us return for a moment to the empty word "I". To introduce meaning into it, I have to differentiate in its semantic space an element of "not-I". I am talking about mutual differentiation and mutual constitution. For example, friends or enemies, by differing from me, constitute me in my relation to them. But to really understand my friend or enemy, I have to understand myself, and to understand myself, I need to understand who my friends and enemies are. If, in order to know x I have to know y and, in turn, in order to know y I have to know x, I beg the question. I turn around in an empty circle, faster and faster, until I can experience the emptiness. The circle is perfect for dancing but few people appreciate it because they think it is a vicious circle, much like tautology, an empty circle. But this emptiness is precisely an imperative of grammar, a prescription of language. It allows us to enter a space beyond death and life. We become Shiva who destroys the world with his dance. When we experience the mutual constitution of contrary terms, meaning disappears and we have a glimpse of what Buddhists call "suchness". This is freedom from meaning, including freedom from such notions as freedom.

Zen Buddhism sees in this freedom the "Great Death" and this is precisely how medical semiotics approaches the issue of death. The "little death" is the biological death of the individual, so called because its importance dwindles in comparison to the death experienced when meaning disappears. The Great Death is the disappearance of our story, our autobiography, not for external but for text-internal reasons. It lies in the nature of words to disappear.

To summarize briefly: medical semiotics views biology as a story within a larger story. *Bios* is a part of *Logos* or, in Socratic terms, *soma* is part of *psyche*. Biological death is part of medical description which, if properly analysed, reveals that the true drama lies in the description through which we view death. It is because *Logos* has a life-and-death structure that we experience *Bios* in those terms. We see life through language; and language is a drama of life and death. Medical semiotics turns biology into a subfield of literature and displaces death from the little scene of a once-in-a-lifetime event into the Great Scene of ontological omnipresence.

2.9. The eternal return of life

If death can be semiotically defined as the death of meaning, what, correspondingly, happens to life? What is life from a semiotic perspective? Life is the eternal return of the same, much like in the case of tautology, of the I am who I am. But what does that mean now, after reviewing the notions of health, disease, and death? We have arrived at the last concept of our inquiry and approach the end of our semiotic reflection. What is life?

We defined health as the movement back and forth from the narrated I to the narrating I, from form to formlessness and back, from history to prehistory, from being to pre-ontology. We noticed a gap in the notion of health, which turned out to be an infinite abyss, between any empirical appearance of health and the normative openness of that notion.

We then defined disease as a process which tends toward the closure of that gap, toward a ready-made identity of those beliefs whose prescriptive destiny we enact. Disease turned out to contain some sado-masochistic components. They consist in the fact that that which makes us suffer, as groups and individuals, is to varying degrees our own doing, insofar as we leave our beliefs unexamined and take the words for granted with which we dramatize our lives. It appears that we can be healthy in conventional terms and yet sick from a semiotic point of view, because we do not let ourselves be pushed by the notion of health toward that point of freedom in which we would be free of even health itself.

Next, we defined death as a movement, internal to language, which naturally moves beyond the definitions of words and sets us free in ways which are unimaginable, since part of the freedom consists in making us free from ourselves. Death is therefore the freedom which is at work in language.

And finally, when it comes to life, what are we saying? What is the semiotic version of life? One thing seems to be clear. Whatever life is, we cannot cling to our notion of life. For when we look over the normative definitions given so far for health, disease, and death, we notice that they have at least one thing in common: they all contain a logical movement which makes them surpass any concrete version of themselves. And this is indeed strange; the fact, namely, that any notion should include its own death as a part of its definition. To know something, I have to go beyond it. This movement seems to be absolute. To get to a notion, I have to be free from it. This is very paradoxical but entirely consistent with the semiotic claim that everything is a sign. In sum, this amounts to saying that nothing can be itself.

If this is true, we know at least that life cannot be itself. It somehow incorporates death, but how? Well it seems that all we have to do at this moment is to apply the law of the mutual constitution of terms in order to see that life and death, by delimiting each other in more or less conventional terms, constitute each other. By themselves, these notions are empty. But the narrating I who enters this dance of words at the moment it entered the scene of language, has to participate in this underlying emptiness of words. If I do, I shall reach freedom. *Wo Es war, soll Ich werden* . Where It was, that is, language, there I shall come to be; that is, I shall be free to be me and not to be me.

We can therefore define life in a first move as a dialogue which is propelled by the attraction of absolute freedom. We are thus led back to the Socratic dialogue with which we began and recognize in the freedom in question the internal absolute freedom of language from itself. But what kind of work is it? It seems that it is comparable to the Great Work, the *Opus Magnum*, of the alchemists, insofar as this work involves a progressive purification or *katharsis* of subjectivity. We can see in this purification a process of progressive liberation from false beliefs.

The work of life, however, is the work of health, the movement back and forth from limitation into freedom and back, from form to formlessness and back, in a Great Circle in which we can recognize the eternal return of the same mystery. It is the mystery of love, of *eros*, not as a mere "subjective" phenomenon, but as the very movement between subject and object. It is the movement of the sentence which, in its most crystalline form, is the movement of tautology; a sentence which proceeds from absolute freedom into any circumstance and back and in this way enacts the pronoun I as an absolute index.

I would like to close this section with the last words of Socrates reported in Plato's dialogue *Phaedo*. Socrates has taken the hemlock, his legs are getting heavy and he has to sit down. Then we read:

> The coldness was spreading about as far as his waist when Socrates uncovered his face, for he had covered it up, and said – they were his last words – Crito, we ought to offer a cock to Asclepius ... (1961: 118a).

At the point of his biological, "little" death, Socrates is bent on enacting the religious ritual of thanking for a cure. A cock is to be sacrificed. According to ancient lore, the cock, at the moment when night turns into day, sees both night and day as one. We can take it, that Socrates, at the very point of biological transition between those states which we call conventionally life and death, was celebrating the absolute freedom from which his speech proceeded and to which it always returned.

3. Guidelines for praxis

In conclusion, I would like to list a few practical consequences which might follow from a semiotic perspective on healing. The most radical dimension of healing is situated in the belief-structure of doctors, nurses, and patients. This belief-structure is in part linguistically accessible and to that extent justifies a semiotic approach to healing. This belief-structure is the target of the therapist's intervention.

The difference of semiotics lies in the fact that the intervention of the therapist does not aim so much at the content of the patient's beliefs, but at the linguistic form in which such beliefs are expressed. This is what I have called the law of the signifier and I have extrapolated two important narratological laws. One is the insurmountable difference and identity between subject and object, or between the narrating I and the narrated I. The other is the fact that meaning arises always in the midst of contradictory and contrary words.

The applicability of these laws to medical practice seems far removed from the immediate concerns of most patients and doctors. This is understandable, because we deal here with the most radical and therefore in many respects most hidden dimension of medicine. Nevertheless, once the relationship of our beliefs to our practice becomes an issue, semiotics can make significant contributions to practice. These contributions are by no means new, as my Plato example shows.

What does an intervention of a semiotically informed perspective look like? Let me say first what kinds of situations lend themselves for a semiotic intervention. The eighteenth century Romantic poet Novalis saw in situations of distress and illness an invitation to examine the meaning of life and death (1983 [1801]). Now this is not exactly your normal medical situation. Mostly people are just concerned with getting over an illness or learning how to cope with it the best they can. There does not seem to be too much room left for what appear to be idle philosophic speculations. But this is no reason why patients cannot be made aware of the fact that what makes them suffer is on the one hand their illness and on the other their perception of their illness. These are two different but interrelated things, and medical semiotics tends to approach illness by way of the perception of illness. That is, it treats illness by treating the perception of illness. Perception and reality are dialectical correlatives.

An intervention in medical semiotics hinges therefore on leading patients from a preoccupation with their illness to a preoccupation with their perception of illness. This reflexive moment is the beginning of semiotic analysis. It is a case of mind over matter but it is quite different from psychosomatic medicine. As I understand psychosomatic medicine, it can show in some cases a physical causal connection between mental and physical problems, as when stress causes intestinal perturbances or high blood pressure. In medical semiotics we have also a causal connection between mind and body, but it is a connection of meaning rather than of physical consequence. This is in line with the fact that medical semiotics does not intervene so much in a given illness as in the conceptual or experiential support of that illness. This leads to an examination of beliefs, ideas, ideals, representations, feelings, and the like, as we saw in the example of Socrates, and such an analysis invariably takes on an aspect of *deconstruction* or decomposition of beliefs.

For example, persons with cancer can and are being led to examine their perception of cancer in order to bring about a perceptual or conceptual change. This is being done in certain hospitals but semiotics could assist here with a refined instrumentarium of how to approach such conceptual and/or perceptual signs. It could initiate a process of de-entification of either the person having cancer or of the cancer as entity itself or of both. Such a process can make the person and/or the cancer literally disappear, albeit not for observers who have no access to the conceptual and emotional decomposition. The deconstruction of disease which medical semiotics initiates here could not be more radical, since the very entities which make up the dramatization of medicine (patient, illness, cure, etc.) are done away with as entities.

Let me just briefly adduce three examples for future discussion. The first example concerns the common sense notion that disease is an outside aggressor. Patients normally perceive their illness as an "it" which attacks them from the outside. They make linguistically a dissociation of "I" and "it". They have the disease, they are not it. Disease is something which affects them, but there is an interesting inside/outside dialectic going on. This gap between the "I" and the disease as an impersonal "it" harbors a deeper truth which we discussed as the impossibility of objectifying the "I". The way patients talk about and experience their disease can be used to make them aware of the fact that whenever we attribute something to the "I", the "I" is and is not the bearer of the attribute. In grammar, this is expressed by the objective case of the predicate. In this way, patients may experience an illness episode as an initiation to the interdict of self-knowledge.

The second example concerns the image of physicians and therapists. They are often perceived as quasi-omnipotent, as subjects who occupy a place of authority, as persons who are supposed to know. This is, as we well know, an ambiguous position. On the one hand it is connected to the unmeasurable benefits of the placebo effect and transference. On the other hand, it is, of course, a kind of deception which reveals a deeper level of the symptom by way of covering it up. This deeper level needs to be uncovered and doctors and patients have to learn how to deal with it. It has to do with facing the lack of self-identity as belonging to the "true nature" of the self. What needs to be uncovered here are our own thought-coverings, i.e. thoughts as coverings of the truth.

In this example, one of the targets of semiotics can be to deconstruct the image of the physician as an agent of authority. This means that while we continue to believe in the art of our physicians, wherever this is possible, and while we continue to trust their dedication, again wherever this is possible, we also learn to see through the entire act of medicine as if it were a kind of trick performed on a sympathetic audience. This seeing through is important, because a semiotic analysis reveals that the entire stage of medicine is a fiction, albeit a very real fiction. But unless one sees it as a fiction, one continues to remain in some kind of iatrogenic or should I say "epistogenic" disease (i.e. disease induced by the physician's beliefs and by our own beliefs).

If it is true that the "I" cannot be predicated insofar as it is a subject, then it is also true that physicians, insofar as they are observable or identifiable agents are precisely to that extent actors in the sense of stage actors. They enact a play written and subscribed to by their beliefs and by our own beliefs. In certain cases it can be very beneficial to lead patients to that obscure place in their own belief-structure, where they write the very story of medicine that they undergo. But this presupposes that therapists have themselves access to that "area" of their mind. Then patients can be taught, sometimes gradually, sometimes almost instantly, that this area is a wide open space, insofar namely as the writing I or the "I" who supports the beliefs cannot be spotted.

Of course, all the various strategies at deconstructing the signifier "I" let us come face to face with our nonsubstantiality as an integral part of the eros of language. And this brings me to my third example, the encounter with death which is central to the medical scene. Semiotics can work out certain steps to integrate death into the living experience of the "I". It is well known that for medical beliefs which tend to identify the "I" unilaterally with the body or with the empirical ego, death is the ultimate victor and therefore defeat for both patients and doctors.

Semiotics may be able to show that this situation is an effect of the fetishism of language. Linguistically induced beliefs remain unexamined and are therefore charged with emotions which make us suffer. The belief in death is a case in point. Upon examination, it reveals itself as the ultimate dramatization of medicine. This means that behind the drama of death is the dramatizer, the narrating I, whose beliefs about death lay out the intellectual and emotional horizon in whose confines he or she is allowed to experience death: truly a magic spell of language.

I do not think we can break this spell, mostly because such a breaking would still be a magic spell of language. But what we can do is to become aware of the spell as a form of enchantment and to enter the song. To hear language sing is to realize that it is always about itself so that if we show patients how to pursue the meaning of the signifier "I", they can begin an infinite journey through language. The main idea here is to show them that each interpretation of the "I" stands in need of another interpretation, and so on, until they are able to affirm the insignificant part of the "I", the "I" as zero signifier, as the one that counts most because it brings them to that open space where it becomes impossible to determine who it is that is dying. Consequently, the grave that we are constantly digging for ourselves with our own beliefs remains wide open and the subject of death can literally not be located and identified.

Note

1. This paper was originally presented at the Semiotics, Psychiatry and Psychoanalysis Conference, Department of Psychiatry, Rush-Presbyterian-St. Luke's Medical Center, March 14, 1987.

References

Baer, Eugen
1988 *Medical semiotics.* Lanham MD: University of America Press.
1989 "Semiotics and medicine", in: Thomas A. Sebeok and Jean Umiker-Sebeok (eds.), 215–269.

Freud, Sigmund
1910 "The antithetical meaning of primal words", S.E. XI, 153. London: The Hogarth Press.
1925 "Negation", S.E. XIX, 235. London: The Hogarth Press.
1933 *New introductory lectures on psychoanalysis.* S.E. XXII. London: The Hogarth Press.

Griffiths, Paul J.
1986 *On being mindless*: Buddhist meditation and the mindbody problem. La Salle IL: Open Court.

Grimstone, A.V. (ed.)
1977 *Two Zen classics.* New York: Weatherhill.

Hegel, Georg Wilhelm Friedrich
1967 *The phenomenology of mind.* [1807] New York: Harper.

Hippocrates
1923 *Hippocrates.* [5th cent. B.C.] 4 vols. New York: Putnam's Sons.

Hume, Robert E.
1971 *The thirteen principal upanishads.* Oxford: Oxford University Press.

Novalis
1983 Das philosophische Werk II Schriften. [1801] Vol. 3. (Edited by Richard Samuel.) Stuttgart: Kohlhammer.

Plato
1961 *The collected dialogues.* [4th cent. B.C.] New York: Bollingen Foundation.

Rosenstock-Huessy, Eugen
1970 *Speech and reality* . Norwich VT: Argo Books.

Sebeok, Thomas A. & Jean Umiker-Sebeok (eds.)
1988 *The Semiotic web 1988.* Berlin–New York: Mouton de Gruyter.

Whitehead, Alfred N.
1967 *Science and the modern world.* New York: Free Press.

The psychodynamic foundation and semiotic reconstruction of psychosomatic medicine

The voice behind the stage:
secret wishes, theory and reality

Thure von Uexküll

Natur und Geist – so spricht man nicht zu Christen.
Deshalb verbrennt man Atheisten,
Weil solche Reden höchst gefährlich sind.

[Nature and Spirit! Words that, in my mind
No Christian man should utter; ‘t is for this
That we burn atheists. Speeches of this kind
Are highly dangerous.]
J.W.v.Goethe, *Faust II*, Lines 4897–4899,
Translation by John Anster, 1864

1. The myth of unprejudiced and disinterested sciences

It is clear that the foundation of psychosomatic medicine cannot be laid by seeking to bridge a "mysterious gap between soma and psyche" (Deutsch 1959). Attempts of this kind are doomed to fail, because their definitions of soma and psyche already contain this gap. Instead, psychosomatic reflection must commence by criticizing the dualistic medicine of bodies without psyche, and psyches without bodies.

Man does not consist of a psycheless body and a bodiless psyche. Conceptions of this sort are the products of theories that construct two incompatible realities. Our question must therefore be: why do we construct these two unrealistic and incompatible realities? And what about the unconscious motives and secret intentions behind these constructions? Why do we hide these motives from ourselves? Answering these questions requires us to critically analyze the interrelationship of theory to reality and practice.

I will try to perform this analysis in two steps: firstly, I will try to investigate the origins and practical relevance of "theories". In the second and essential step of my investigation I will try to view this problem from the opposite perspective; namely, by discussing its relations to modern medicine. In other words, I will look for the "theories" behind medical practice and constructions of medical reality. For only by understanding the reasons for the development of our present system of somatological and psychological medicine can we hope to properly approach the foundation of a holistic, psychosomatic or bio-psycho-somatic medicine.

In the course of this discussion it will become clear that the traditional concept of sciences as a disinterested and unprejudiced proceeding is but a myth. We always knew about our need for theories in the description of natural phenomena. But today we have to accept Wittgenstein's (1953) reminder that all human descriptions are but tools adapting phenomena for the specific use we intend to make of them.

2. The genetic question: why and when are theories created?

Animals do not require theories for their orientation in nature. Why do humans need theories? What happened to us, creating this necessity? Not wanting to respond to these questions in metaphysical terms, we have to resort to the evolution of man. And given the scarce and fragmentary accounts of phylogenetic material, we have to proceed by investigating our ontogenetic past; that is, our early childhood.

Freud has made some important remarks on this subject. I quote here from his paper on "The two fundamental principles of psychological events" (1911: 229):[1]

> In order to integrate the psychological relevance of external reality into the concept of our thoughts, we thus have to examine the developing relation of the neurotic, and of *man in general* to reality. In a psychology based upon psycho-analysis we have grown accustomed to start off with unconscious emotional events ... The governing principle of these primary processes is easily recognized; we have called it the pleasure-pain-principle (or simply the pleasure-principle). These emotional tendencies strive to achieve pleasure; from acts attached with pain, they refrain. [Emphasis added]

Freud then delineates the birth of rational thought and its concept of "reality" as emerging from these early primary processes. Reaching back to models developed in his 1900 book on "Dream theory" he writes (1911: 229):

> I suppose an incipient disturbance of the primary psychic peace by strong internal demands. In these cases, whatever was needed is simply 'created' by hallucination, a process observable in the same way every night when we dream ... (Since this cannot bring about the expected satisfaction, the psychic apparatus was compelled to decide): it had *to imagine the conditions of*

> *external reality and to aim at changing this reality.* A new principle of psychic activity was thus introduced. [Emphasis added]

I will skip over the question of why Freud could not fully conceptualize the revolutionary thought of a reality, constructed by the actions and effects of the pleasure-principle on our mind. He still accepted the nineteenth century dogma postulating a given reality of things in themselves (*Ding an sich*).

Having witnessed the revolution of quantum physics in natural sciences, we are more apt to understand Freud's message today as follows: what we call the "real conditions of external reality" is nothing but a construction, forced upon our imagination by the pleasure principle. While sketching the scenarios in which we search for the tours and detours necessary for the achievement of goals inaccessible to direct approach, our imagination consequently borrows its creative capacities from the modes of thought and wishful thinking habitual to our dreams.

This creative capacity, taken from the model of hallucinatory wish-fulfillment in dreams, we call "phantasy". The term is derived from the Greek *phainesthai*, meaning 'let come into apparition'. And in order to let something come into appearance, phantasy produces what the Greeks called *theoria*. The Greek *theorein* means 'to see', in the sense of scheming stages on which we – like in theaters, the places of seeing – act as actors in the imaginary scenarios designed by the pleasure-principle. In their dictionary of psychoanalytic terms, Laplanche and Pontalis (1972) define imagination as the capacity to outline imaginary scenarios. These scenarios themselves – in which the subject is present – then represents the fulfillment of a wish, more or less distorted by the actions of our defense mechanisms.

The theories by which we frame our scientific realities now are – and this is the main thesis of my paper – originally dreams, equally dependent on unconscious wishes and drives, forcing us to seek methods for their fulfillment and satisfaction. They, too, demonstrate the compulsion enacted on our mind by the pleasure-principle. And the persuasive power of scientific realities derives from their ability to fulfill the demands of the pleasure-principle (and not from their alleged exactness and realistic truth). The content-reality of scientific theories thus is borrowed from the reality of those passions which Freud in *Beyond the pleasure principle* (1920) described as the darkest and least accessible realm of the psyche.

3. Medicine as an example of the power of the unconscious in medical-scientific theories

Questioning the origins of scientific theories has led us to an answer contradictory to all our traditional learning about theories. Does it not seem virtually absurd to claim that the realities of, say, chemistry and physics, commonly regarded as completely devoid of all subjective contaminations, borrow their conceptions of reality from passions hidden in our unconscious wishes?

I will leave this question unanswered for the moment. Instead of jumping to a premature conclusion I will insert a second step into my analysis: an investigation of the realities created by sciences, and the theories applied in their construction. It seems to me that the realities of medicine are an appropriate example for an investigation of this kind. For its dualistic contradictions plainly invite an analysis of its theoretical foundations. In this analysis we will gradually realize that our emotional tendencies contradictory to social rules are not the only objects of repression. We will also detect that we are capable of collectively repressing the cognitive principles, organizing and determining thought and practise in science. It is this double repression that helps us to hide our irrationalities behind the facade of what we believe to be scientific rationality.

On the following pages I will attempt a questioning of the realities in medicine as these relate to leading principles behind the interaction of doctors and patients. At the same time I will look for hidden tendencies, secretly influencing these leading principles.

3.1. Theory, instrument and reality

Before entering the analysis of these realities, however, I first have to mention a basic precondition for the analysis of the theories behind our realities. Theories frame scenarios of routes leading us to the achievement of goals, inaccessible to direct realization. This framing is greatly influenced by the fact that these routes have to be drafted by changing our respective environments. This adds enormous significance to the instruments at our disposal for the modification of these environments.

Nature had endowed man with two main instruments for accomplishing changes in his environments: hand and word. Their different phylogenetic history is reflected in their individual ontogenesis as revealed by modern developmental psychology (e.g., Piaget and Inhelder 1977, Winnicott 1971, Mahler, Pine & Bergman 1980, Hoffer 1964/65, Hofer 1981). Motor activity, and especially the motorics of the hand, dominate the imagination of the child up to an age of approximately 20 months. The hand becomes the first major instrument of changing a reality which – at this period – remains still a part of the child.

From that time on, as Piaget (1975) has shown, an imagination exploiting the creative capacities of dreaming begins to dominate the child's mind. Scenarios of an internal imagination occur together with scenarios of external reality. And within this internal imagination behavior begins to be modified by 'hypothetical acting' (*Probehandeln*, Freud), that is, by thought. From this stage on, the acquisition of language, and hence the word as instrument, attains an ever increasing importance for our construction of an outside world. The introduction of language can be interpreted as the introduction of the creative capacities of dreaming into our conscious imagination and thought (Edelson 1972). Words thus become the second major instrument changing reality.

3.2. Paradigm and diagnosis

There are general theories depicting open scenarios with many alternative possibilities of problem-solving. Thomas Kuhn (1962) has proposed the term "paradigm" for these theories. According to Kuhn, a scientific paradigm exemplifies a solution for a problem hitherto unsolved. The paradigm then becomes an example for the handling of similar or related scientific problems. Finally, it enters the lectures, textbooks and prescriptions for experimental and teaching practice of the students of the respective disciplines.

Paradigms are used as a general example for the specific theories developed within the frame of the sciences they found. In medicine these specific theories are called "diagnoses". Diagnoses outline limited scenarios with well defined rules for the interaction of doctors and patients. I hold that modern medicine is cleaved by the existence of two different, mutually exclusive paradigms with two different kinds of diagnoses. Medicine hence is split into two different scientific concepts constituting two different scientific realities. One of these paradigms founds the so-called "scientific" medicine. This mainstream branch of medicine is based on the application of the physical sciences. I prefer to call it biotechnical medicine. The second of these paradigms constitutes the so-called "psychological" medicine, which I prefer to call psychotherapeutic medicine.

I will now try to analyze these two realities of modern medicine by revealing their different paradigmatic theories. In a later stage of my analysis I will try to detect unconscious wishes (that is, fantasies of the pleasure-principle or of passion) hidden within these theories. For only an unprejudiced comparison of these two realities and their conscious as well as their unconscious backgrounds enables us to solve the problem of a "holistic", psychosomatic medicine. I begin by analyzing the pragmatic system of biotechnical medicine.[2]

3.3. The pragmatic system of biotechnical medicine

3.3.1. The paradigm of the machine

The leading principle constituting the reality of biotechnical medicine, founding a pragmatic system of diagnosis acting as stage directions for doctors and patients, is derived from the physics of the nineteenth century. At that time, the paradigm of the machine as a solution for problems hitherto unsolved by the instrument of the hand, began its victorious march through the civilized world. By transferring this model onto the body-concept a well differentiated scheme of orientation for manual intervention into the human body was developed. Simpler forms of this model certainly date back to very ancient epochs and probably constituted, in different variations, components of all medical systems as manual interventions into the body of patients carried out by healing shamans or practitioners.

Irrespective of already being defined or not, the common denominator of all these systems is the concept "mechanic cause". This concept interprets the internal events of the body as causal interdependencies. Within this model it becomes possible to imagine that the same events can be produced by manual interventions. C. von Ferber (1971) has drawn our attention to the connection of the rise of modern industrialism and the development of modern biotechnical medicine. And it is this association that helps us to understand the stubborn maintenance of this basic concept of manual intervention in modern medicine, despite its dynamic development into a highly complex theoretical system.

The ever increasing sophistication of direct manual interventions, due to technical devices, or of indirect, pharmaceutical interventions, due to the progress in modern pharmacology, compelled medicine to differentiate its model of the body. This differentiation in turn further stimulated the sophistication of direct and indirect interventional techniques. Thus evolved the global and impressive system of modern medicine, defining the human body as an ever more complex physico-biochemical machine.

Disease now is defined as a localized breakdown in a technical plant which, despite its complexity, is ready for successful technical surveillance by the help of the machine-model as a general scheme of orientation. Diagnoses become schemes for specific technical breakdowns, enclosing the technical directions for the handling of short-circuits, leaking pipes, transport jams and other problems. Like a technician, localizing, planning and enacting the repair of a technical breakdown in a car, TV set or a computer with the help of a circuit diagram, the modern physician attempts to localize, define and "cure" the technical breakdowns of the human body – i.e., valvular defects in the heart, ulcers in the stomach or enzyme dysfunctions in tissues – with the help of specific technical (surgical or pharmaceutical) interventions.

The technical terminology of physics, chemistry and biochemistry provides an adequate language for this pragmatic system. Since one cannot talk with, only about machines, more traditional forms of communicating with patients become "unscientific" and dysfunctional within this model. Consequently, communication between doctors and patients develops into an exchange of preconceived questions and preinterpreted replies, imitating the model of the technician's check-up list.

The final stage of this development is marked by the replacement of the clinical interview with the use of computerized questionnaires.

Doctors and patients are similarly affected by this development. The more conclusively the patient is reduced to a machine, the more his doctor turns into a technician and his work into a technical procedure. The personalities of patients and physicians evaporate from the relationship between clients and doctors. Finally, the doctor so completely vanishes behind medical apparati that he mutates into the robot shown standing at the bedside of futuristic hospitals in the medical caricatures of our time.

It is crucial to see this development not as a mere accident of medical-scientific history, but as the culmination of a central tendency inherent in the machine-theory of man. Biotechnical medicine has inherited Lammetries' eighteenth century call for *l'homme-machine* as one of the first impressive realizations of unconscious omnipotence phantasies of early childhood. The utopian concept of a *Brave new world*, that is, a society fully manipulated and "liberated" by its own technique, is a hallucination of the pleasure-principle. And the drive of biotechnical medicine towards an ever more conclusive perfection derives its internal dynamic from this very source.

The German psychoanalyst H. E. Richter (1987) speaks of the "God-complex" of modern man. In this system of systematic omnipotence, disease is defined as a societal deficit in technical perfection and medicine as the societal agent endowed with the task to overcome this deficit. The irrational background of the cognitive principles in biotechnical medicine became a victim of repression.

3.3.2. Critical interlude

The theses put forward in this paper sharply contradict the common opinions on science and medicine. They contradict, moreover, the palpable success of biotechnical medicine and its principal theories in the conquest of nature. Until recently this success was indeed overwhelming; and the scientific and medical pride attained within this story of success dismissed all critical reflection as the pure product of romanticizing hostility against science and technique.

This general feeling has changed in the last decades. The pride has – at least partly – vanished and we begin to realize the cost of our spectacular technical success: a destruction of natural resources that has reached dangerous dimensions, leaving the majority of scientists and technicians without a suitable answer. Theoretical discussions of the responsibility of scholars for the results of their research have suddenly gained practical relevance in light of complications of nuclear technology and genetic engineering, concrete problems widely known to today's public.

This "failure of success" has turned technological optimism into pessimism. The disappointment of irrational desires caused by the contemporary ecological and political crises thus contains once again the danger of a generalized, iconoclastic hostility against science. We are confronted with a problem whose indissolubility is the very problem: researchers still reject any responsibility for the practical application of their "purely scientific" research dedicated to truth and nothing but truth. They refuse any political control as a violation of the scientist's "freedom of research". But the real problem lies in the incapability of scientists and politicians to reliably predict the ecological, social and political consequences of applied science and new techniques. Neither long-term nor long-distance effects can be calculated in the short time spans usually given for political and scientific decision making.

Insoluble contradictions of this kind indicate deep-rooted dissociations and conflicts. Bateson (1972) has traced the origin of today's problems back to our "diseased epistemology", to the "epistemological fallacies of occidental civilization". According to him, Darwin was a victim of this disease while constructing his theory of natural selection. While regarding the species as the "natural entity of survival" in a hostile and mercilessly selecting environment it escaped his attention that the "natural entity of survival in the real biological world consists of the organism and its environment" (1972: 483). Today, Bateson adds, "we learn the bitter lesson that an organism destroying its environment destroys itself" (1972: 483). Our "diseased epistemology" is the expression of our blindness for the irrational and unconscious desires hidden within our scientific theories. This is the epistemological background for analyzing the problem of the responsibility of research and our inability to cope with it. But what about the basic paradigms and leading principles of psychological medicine?

3.4. The pragmatic system of psychological medicine

3.4.1. The paradigm of the "psychic apparatus"

Biotechnical medicine's definitions of disease and health do not fulfill most people's expectations of a humane medical treatment. But this inability is not a product of inhumane physicians. It is the dominating pragmatic system that forces its members to behave, think and act in a manner functionally appropriate to its basic theories.

At the time of Freud's inaugurating attempt to treat patients not with hands (or hand-related instruments) but with words, the success of biotechnical medicine and the belief in infinite progress by an ever advancing technique had already become a religion. Using his new methods, Freud himself believed that he did nothing but to continue the practice of technical medicine by the usage of different means. His term "psychic apparatus" documents this well. But soon it became obvious that Freud's diagnostic and therapeutic method of talking with patients had initiated another paradigm in medicine, in contrast to the paradigm of the machine. Within this new paradigm "psyche" is not defined as an apparatus or mechanism, but rather as an entity we could describe, in today's language, as an "autopoetic system" – i.e., a system with a time-related structure as the result of a gradual socialization of biological needs.

Thus a new model of orientation for physicians took shape. Comparable to the annual rings in a tree by which the gardener can date the developmental difficulties of a plant, the physician can localize the cause of an emotional disease in a specific phase of his patient's psycho-sexual development. Furthermore, the model allows a dynamic interpretation in the sense that it enables the physician to imagine various elements of the psychic structure deriving from different phases of emotional development to be simultaneously active in the patient's psyche. Instead of the spatial scheme of orientation in biotechnical medicine, Freud's model presents a chronological scheme of orientation. Instead of localizing sources of disease for the intervention of the physician's hand, disease is now defined as a defect in the *Zeitgestalt* ('time structure') within the socialization-history of an individual. Disturbances of this kind cannot be treated by manual interventions into patients' bodies, but by talking with them. Talking attains a fundamental significance in psychotherapeutic medicine parallel to the importance of manual intervention in biotechnical medicine. Talking is subject to a gradually developing sophistication of diagnostic and therapeutic methods applied to ever more specific concepts of emotional disease.

The new paradigm again acts as a general concept for the diagnosis of specific diseases. Far from being restricted to the merely phenomenological description of typical behavioral disturbances, these diagnoses now appear as well defined defects in the *Zeitgestalt* of an individual's socialized formation accessible to etiological and pathogenetic explanations. And – at least in principle – this new concept of disease resulting from a socialization-defect in the formation-history of the psychic system opens the gate for a new approach to therapy. This new paradigm also organizes and defines the rules for the interaction of doctors and clients; and again the roles of physicians and patients are complementary.

3.4.2. The psyche as the creative organizor of the relation between organism and environment

We have observed how the paradigm of the machine developed into a model interpreting the body as a counterplay to the physician's hand. Anatomy is the science describing the different structures of this "handy" body. Anatomy hence enables us to vividly imagine the physical events within the body during the physician's direct and indirect manual intervention. The relative irrelevance of language and speech for this enterprise does not take us by surprise.

We have then observed how the paradigm of time-structured disease developed into a model interpreting the psyche as a counterplay of the physician's words. But it still remains to describe the specific mode by which this inpalpable medium dubbed *psyche* turns into a "palpable substance" affected, altered, amplified by words. Freud has called this substance *libido*. He developed a differentiated model in which this substance organizes through specific phases into a highly complex structure. His successors have further extended and sophisticated this model. Given this, my precis of the Freudian model as the time-structured concept of the historical fate of individual instinctual impulses may seem grossly oversimplified. But still the main paradigmatic factor of Freudian theory lies in the socializing (i.e., curative or destructive) power of language. But in order to receive an answer to the question how this substance and its being influenced by speech should be imagined we have to go one step further. We have to acknowledge the collectively repressed fact that every one of us inhabits his own private and personally owned individual reality. Not only every pain, but every sensation, emotion or thought is a strictly private event. Nobody can feel another's pain or sensation; nobody can see the other's colors or think his thoughts. This private world of the individual represents his environment, his *Umwelt*. In other words, this *Umwelt* represents the environment which, as Bateson emphasizes, constitutes together with our body the "true unit of biological survival".

This private world of individual reality not only is inescapably connected to our body; it developed in constant interaction with us in the medium of communication with mother, family and peer or professional groups. This medium of communication is the sphere within which we have learned that our private sensations, emotions, wishes and thoughts only gained significance and relevance when being named; that is, once they were integrated into the verbal and nonverbal semiotic systems of our family (or its surrogates and successors).

Signs of all kinds were the thread by which we learnt to weave our subjective impressions as a protective tissue around our body. And since these signs are – at a very early stage, around the beginning of the second year – reinforced by the threads of the semiotic system of language, we are entitled to say that our psyche weaves the tissue of individual reality with the "threads of words". Within this tissue words have a connecting as well as a disconnecting function. Not surprisingly, words can also act as destroyers of this tissue (viz. Harley Shands [1971] who wrote about the war with words). For this tissue is the substrate on which and in which words enact their many-sided and manifold influence.

3.4.3. The motives behind the reality of psychotherapeutic medicine

What about the result of our analyzing the different realities of dualistic medicine? Could this analysis possibly help us to understand the reasons behind the construction of two mutually exclusive realities? And, moreover, could it help us to find a solution for this dualistic dilemma?

The motive behind the paradigm of psychotherapeutic medicine is rooted in the obligation of every society to guarantee its younger citizens the chance of intact socialization, letting them grow into fully accepted members of their native societal system. Viewed from the task of the best socialization for the greatest number, disease then appears as a socially caused defect in socialization that has to be compensated for by medicine. From the psychodynamic point of view, motives of this kind are related to the Oedipal phase of psychic development. In this phase triadic (or more) person-relationships develop and the threefold structure of occidental language (with subject, object and verb) begins to dominate the phantasy and imaginative activities of the child.

In contrast, the motive behind the theories and promises of biotechnical medicine stems from earlier stages of psychodynamic growth. There we are confronted with the basic problems of liberation from the primary objects of the symbiotic stage and their seemingly unlimited promise of security and protection. The "bad mother" of this stage is the mother that fails to meet the desires of her infant instantaneously; resentful fantasies of infantile omnipotence are the answer to events of this type.

The main mistake of psychotherapeutic medicine consists in the unreflected acceptance of the body-concepts of biotechnical medicine with the result of dualistic thinking; notwithstanding the fact that attempts of a critical evaluation can be traced back already to Sandor Ferenczi's writings. This criticism was later further developed and differentiated by Michael Balint (1965), Melanie Klein (1972), D.W. Winnicott (1971), and W.R. Bion (1962). But despite all these critical efforts, the main dualistic dilemma remained untouched. The social motives in psychotherapeutic medicine initially came into conflict with the leading ideologies of contemporary society, but they were not to be repressed as were the phantasies of omnipotence, whose repression gave the theories of biotechnical medicine their dynamic impact. The "socially produced unconsciousness" (M. Erdheim 1982) was much easier to overcome than the repression of the earlier omnipotence-phantasies, the result of which was the whole occidental tradition since Plato.

It is no wonder that attempts to integrate the social dimensions of disease into psychoanalysis (Erik Erikson 1957; V. von Weizsäcker 1986; A. Mitscherlich 1966, and others) were by far more successful than efforts to overcome the resistance against the unveiling of the omnipotent phantasies that stem from the much earlier phase in which rational thought was invented as a "new principle of psychic activity".

3.4.4. The voice behind the stage

Considering Bateson's thesis of our "diseased epistemology" it seems of eminent importance to investigate the developmental history of man's epistemological capacities, i.e., the ontogenesis of his thinking. The writings of D.W. Winnicott on the development of the object-concept are very important in this regard. They have extended, criticized and complemented the Freudian developmental theory of the reality-principle in its positivistic version. Winnicott's genetic epistemology will be the key to solving the philosophical and scientific problem inherent in the crucial terms *object* and *objectivity*, whose clarification is indispensable for all the physical and psychological sciences.

In this space, I can only give a few hints about this phenomenon. According to Winnicott, the dramatic history of the mutually dependent development of subject and object can be described by four key terms: object-relationship; object-usage and object-destruction; object-annihilation. All these terms reflect different aspects of time whose rise and fall, development and durance, are no abstract rational problems within Winnicott's theory but the passionate experiences of living phenomena. They reflect life with all its abysses of birth, disease, dying and death. In this history of human time – or this concept of time as the essence of human history – the possibility of failing is deeply involved. The possible failure of emotional and rational development and the pathology of our epistemology as the instrument for constructing the world in which we live is the dramatic core of Winnicott's thought – and the key to its centrality to the discussion of biotechnical medicine and science.

Individual human history thus can be described as a "chain of developments" between object-relation and object-usage: it begins with the "subjective creation" of the newborn's first object, the mother's breast. In this constellation subject and object still form an entity (of "survival"):

> In clinical terms: two babies are feeding at the breast. One is feeding on the self, since the breast and the baby have not yet become (for the baby) separate phenomena (D.W. Winnicott 1971: 89).

At the next level the first object is destroyed:

> This change (from relating to usage) means that the subject destroys the object ... In other words "subject relates to object" becomes "subject destroys object" (as it becomes external) ... That is, the subject's perception of the ob-

> ject as an external phenomenon, not as a projective entity, is in fact the recognition of it as an entity in its own right (D.W. Winnicott 1971: 89, 90).

If everything goes all right, the position of object-survival follows after the destruction of the object by the subject. However, the object can, but must not survive. Thus the possibility of failing and pathological development come into sight. For only a surviving object can be "used" by the subject:

> By "use" I do not mean "exploitation". As analysts, we know what it is like to be used ... they (the patients, subjects) can use the objects and they can use us and analysis, just as they have used their parents and their siblings and their homes (D.W. Winnicott 1971: 94).

The two other main Winnicottian terms, destruction and annihilation, emphasize the affective significance of time. Destruction in this context has a positive meaning (as in Goethe's famous demand: die to be born). The subjective object is destroyed and thus put "outside the area of the subject's omnipotent control" (1971: 89). The second term, annihilation, however has a negative connotation; it simply means 'no hope' (death) (1971: 93).

Any possible pathological development has to be understood in the light of the fact that the position of object-usage can be reached only if the object shall survive:

> In other words, because of the survival of the object, the subject may now have started to live a life in the world of objects, and so the subject stands to gain immeasurably; but the price has to be paid in the acceptance of the ongoing destruction in the unconscious phantasy relative to object-relating. Let me repeat. This is a position that can be arrived at by the individual in early stages of emotional growth only through the actual survival of cathected subjects that are at the time in process of becoming destroyed because real, becoming real because destroyed (being destructible and expendable) (D.W. Winnicott 1971: 90).

And the object in turn can only survive if it does not take revenge for having been destroyed. "Vengeance" is another crucial term for Winnicott:

> From now on the subject says "Hullo object", "I destroyed you", "I love you"; "You have value for me because of your survival of my destruction of you", "While I am loving you I am all the time destroying you in (uncon-

scious) phantasy". Here phantasy begins for the individual. The subject can now use the object that has survived (D.W. Winnicott 1971: 90).

Transposing Winnicott's concepts to our problem, we can venture to say that it is the main problem of occidental culture to destroy objects in a manner that allows their survival. We fail to give them leave from our omnipotent control and we fail to accept their right to develop into beings of individual and proper self-control. So objects – in the imagination of most philosophers and scientists – remain potentially "manipulated objects". Objects of this kind cannot be used, but only exploited and abused.

This conceptualization is connected to another psychological fact: to take revenge or not to take revenge is not only a problem of the destroyed objects but also of the subjects destroying the objects in their unconscious phantasy. The frustration-tolerance of the subject decides whether and when it experiences the loss of object-control as the revenge of the object for having been destroyed. Bion (1962) has put forward that the frustration-tolerance of our human epistemological faculty is generally overpowered by the task of accepting objects as living and independent phenomena. He argues that we tend to resort to pseudo-solutions of this problem by claiming the reality of the non-living as the reality of life.

The problem is threatening indeed: destruction always includes and approaches annihilation, and annihilation of the object always potentially includes annihilation of the subject. Given this, the fear of being annihilated is generated. And this very fear, I finally conclude, turns out to be the "voice behind the stage" in the theories of the physical sciences depicting the scenario of a reality from which sources and sites of fear are systematically excluded.

This systematic exclusion of fear is the reason behind our inability to release objects from the realm of omnipotent manipulation. And this is why living time has to vanish, for this is the dangerous period in which objects may change their minds and shapes beyond our control. In other words, the price paid by science for the ever more intelligent control of objects is their very life and vitality.

Newton founded classical physics by eliminating the irreversibility of time – and consequently life. For time indeed is irreversible in the processes of evolution, growth, development and vanishing of life (see Prigogine & Stengers 1981). The same goal is attempted by the paradigm of the machine in medicine: negating the irreversibility of time in disease and dying. For a machine is always an object of potentially perfect repair and in this process of technical repair the vector from rise to fall can be reversed to the direction from fall to rise. Final conclusiveness and non-reversibility are invalid, even non-existent, for the virtually eternal "life" of the machine.

The failing last act in the drama of the subject's way to object-usage and "matured love" (M. Balint 1965) thus could be the etiology of the "diseased epistemology of occidental science." Descartes did not invent dualism. Rather, he was a victim of the same epistemology. Nevertheless, two post-Cartesian developments have added their share to the process that included our bodies among the objects unable to survive their destruction by science. Our bodies thus degenerated into objects of technical manipulations: 1) our inability to read the signs given by objects that have remained beings in their own right with self-controlled vitality; 2) the replacement of this inability by the experience of anatomy and physiology that the body of the corpse is limitlessly subjected to manipulation. The problem of bodies and souls thus became a problem of corpses and souls. Hand and word (i.e., signs), our instruments for intervention in reality, and the unconscious wishes and desires behind our scientific theories are the background for our dualistic medicine for bodies without souls and souls without bodies.

4. The problem of a psychosomatic medicine and its semiotic solution

Contrasting the two basic paradigms hand, i.e., mechanical cause for biotechnical medicine, and word, i.e., linguistic cause for psychotherapeutic medicine, the problem of a psychosomatic medicine can be seen more clearly: we have to find a common denominator for hand and word. Looking for phenomena present in everyday medical practise and unrelated to either of these systems we happen to meet a widely misunderstood phenomenon: the *placebo*. The Latin *placebo* means 'I will please' and is generally used to describe positive (and negative) side effects of medical intervention (usually pharmaceutical but also surgical or manual) inaccessible to anatomical or pharmacological explanations. We speak of a "suggestive effect", but no one has a clear concept what this wants to say.

We will get closer to a solution to our problem when taking two facts into consideration. 1) Living systems do not react to physical or chemical stimuli like mechanisms; rather they code all incoming stimuli into signs; that is, they are responding to signs. 2) All signs are "two-sided" (Sebeok 1976). They consist of a chemical or physical "carrier" and a signification, a message or information for the receiver.

Words, too, are – as are all signs – "two-sided". Physically they consist of waves in the air causing mechanical effects in the ear; semantically they consist of a signification, message or information that has to be decoded by the receiver. All physician-manual interventions are in this sense two-sided, too. Direct surgical procedures as well as indirect pharmaceutical interventions have mechanical effects (of an anatomical, physical or chemical type) as well as significations for the system they are acting upon. They, too, are signs conferring specific information.

It is fatally one-sided to focus only on the mechanical or the semantic aspects of disease. All doctors' activities – from initial handshake, clinical interview, physical examination, or prescription of a drug to surgical procedure or psychotherapeutic talk – clearly are two-sided. Although to a vastly different degree, they have mechanical effects on the body of the patient and they bear significations that are consciously or rather mostly unconsciously decoded by the patient. The physician thus has to take the semiotic aspect of all his actions into account.

Given this, the placebo effect does not appear as a marginal phenomenon suggesting the ineffectivity of medical procedures, but rather as the paradigm of a "holistic" medicine; for it contains the key for the self-assembly of the units of life and survival consisting of organisms and environment (Bateson 1972). *Placebo* means 'I will please(or displease)'. This represents the assignment of meaning to a sign; that is, the coding of relevant parts of the environment into vehicles for the semantic connection between the organism and the fluctuant contents of his surrounding reality.

A holistic medicine following this paradigm would never relinquish biotechnical medicine, for it defines and identifies the vehicles and their respective mechanical impact on the biological receptors of living systems. Biotechnical medicine thus creates the preconditions for the investigation of coding functions that organize the transformation of different vehicles into different signs. It would be the task of a biosemiotic medicine to analyze the interaction of the manifold semiotic processes at the levels of cells, tissues, organs as well as at the level of the organism in interaction with the environment. This biosemiotic medicine also would have to investigate the translating processes between the different levels of integration forming the base for upward and downward effects between the levels of cells and the level of social systems. Medicine is – so I could summarize my account – a semiotic science in which the realities of biotechnical and psychotherapeutic medicine yet have to be integrated within the frame of an encompassing reality of sign-relations.

Notes

1. I owe the knowledge of these interdependencies to E. Grassi (1989).
2. The following pages are partly taken from T. von Uexküll (1980).

References

Antonowsky, A.
1987 "The salutogenetic perspective: toward a new view of health and illness", *Advances* 4.1, 47–55.
Balint, Michael
1965 *Primary love and psychoanalytic technique*. London: Tavistock Publications.
Bateson, Gregory
1972 "Pathologies of epistemology", in: *Steps to an ecology of mind*. New York: Chandler Publishing. (German translation: *Ökologie des Geistes*, Frankfurt am Main: Suhrkamp 1985.)
Bion, W.R.
1962 *Learning from experience*. London: William Heinemann Medical Books. H. Karnac Ltd.
Deutsch, F.
1959 *On the mysterious leap from the mind to the body*. London: International Universities Press.
Edelson, Marshall
1972 "Language and dreams: *The interpretation of dreams* revisited", *The Psychoanalytic Study of the Child* 27: 203–282.
Erdheim, M.
1982 *Die gesellschaftliche Produktion von Unbewußtheit*. Frankfurt am Main: Suhrkamp.
Erikson, Erik H.
1957 *Kindheit und Gesellchaft*. Zürich: Pan-Verlag.
Ferber, C.von
1971 "Die Verständigung zwischen Arzt und Patient", *Der praktische Arzt* 8, 888–902.
Freud, Sigmund
1900 *Die Traumdeutung*. G.W. 2/3. London: Imago Publishing Co. S.E. IV & V. London: The Hogarth Press.
1911 "Formulierungen über die zwei Prinzipien des psychischen Geschehens", G.W. 8, 229. London: Imago Publishing Co. S.E. XII, 213. London: The Hogarth Press.
1920 *Beyond the pleasure principle*. G.W. 13, 1 London: Imago Publishing Co. S.E. XVIII, 1. London: The Hogarth Press.
Grassi, E.
1989 "Freud's pleasure-principle as a base for contemporary realistic philos-

ophy", in: *Ur-Sprung-An-Spruch der Natur in der Lust*. München: Züricher Gespräche, W. Fink Verlag,

Hofer, M.A.
1981 *The roots of behavior*. San Francisco CA: Freeman.

Hoffer, W.
1964/65 "Mund, Hand und Ich-Integration", *Psyche* XVIII, 81-88. (English original: *The Psychoanalytic Study of the Child* 3/4. 1949.)

Iappe, G. & C. Nedelmann (eds.)
1980 *Zur Psychoanalyse der Objektbeziehungen*. Stuttgart: Frommann und Holzboog.

Klein, Melanie
1972 *Das Seelenleben des Kindes und andere Beiträge*. Reinbek: Rowohlt.

Kuhn, Thomas
1962 *The structure of scientific revolutions*. Chicago IL: University of Chicago Press.

Laplanche, Jean & J.-B. Pontalis
1972 *Das Vokabular der Psychoanalyse*. Frankfurt am Main: Suhrkamp.

Mahler, Margaret S., Fred Pine, & Anni Bergman
1980 *Die psychische Geburt des Menschen*. Frankfurt am Main: Fischer.

Mitscherlich, A.
1966 "Die Krankheiten der Gesellschaft und die psychosomatische Medizin", *Werke* I. Frankfurt am Main: Suhrkamp.

Piaget, Jean
1975 "Der Aufbau der Wirklichkeit beim Kinde", [1937] *Gesammelte Werke* II. Stuttgart: Klett.

Piaget, Jean & Bärbel Inhelder
1977 *Die Psychologie des Kindes*. Frankfurt am Main: Fischer.

Prigogine, I. & I. Stengers
1981 *Dialog mit Natur*. München: Piper.

Richter, H.E.
1987 *Der Gotteskomplex*. Reinbek: Rowohlt.

Sebeok, Thomas A.
1976 *Contribution to a doctrine of signs*. Bloomington IN: Indiana University Press.
1978 *The sign and its masters*. Austin TX: University of Texas Press.

Shands, Harley
1971 *The war with words*. The Hague: Mouton.

Uexküll, Jakob von
1928 *Theoretische Biologie* 2. Auflage Berlin: Springer, Neudruck. Frankfurt am Main: Suhrkamp. 1973.

Uexküll, Thure von
1980 "Das Problem der Entsprechung von Rollen und Gegenrollen bei Arzt und Patient", in: G. Iappe & C. Nedelmann (eds.), 37–73.
Weizsächer, Viktor von
1986 *Gesammelte Schriften*. Frankfurt am Main: Suhrkamp.
Winnicott, Donald W.
1971 *Playing and reality*. New York: Basic Books.
Wittgenstein, Ludwig
1953 *Philosophical investigations*. Oxford: Blackwell.

A semiotic approach to alexithymia

Phillip S. Epstein

Introduction

By way of introduction, I would like first to provide a brief description of the origins of this chapter and the work that it describes. Throughout my years of clinical experiences as an academic psychiatrist, I had become deeply impressed by the basic and obvious fact that much of our time as psychotherapists or psychopharmacotherapists is spent in assisting our patients to deal with poorly identified, understood, expressed or regulated feeling states. I was, therefore, impressed by Peter Sifneos' discussion, presented during a visit to the Rush Medical School's department of psychiatry, of his work on *alexithymia*, a term he coined for the condition of being 'without the words for feelings'.

As a consequence of his visit, I formed a small informal group to begin study of this intriguing concept that promised to address a core issue in my work. My background had prepared me to view emotions in terms of neurophysiology and psychodynamics; Sifneos' research added a new emphasis on the labeling and communication of those feelings. Subsequently, Arnold Goldberg and Bonnie Litowitz asked me to assist in the planning and development of a conference on semiotics, psychiatry and psychoanalysis, exposing me formally for the first time to the discipline of semiotics. As we prepared for the conference and I learned more about semiotics, it seemed to me that a semiotically informed clinical theory could contribute significantly to psychiatry in general and to the problem of alexithymia in particular. Further clinical research in psychopharmacotherapy and alexithymia, as well as continued study of semiotics, has left me even more convinced. So much of what we are concerned with as clinicians and researchers reduces to problems of sign or signal definition, transmission, reception and interpretation. For example, the brain is continuously sending, receiving and processing signals about its internal states. Perhaps a person with alexithymia is having difficulty in reading his or her own affects as signals, identifying feelings with signs, and therefore is unable to communicate effectively about emotions to others. One advantage, then, of semiotics is that it seems to offer the possibility of providing a more effective way to articulate and relate both the neurobiological underpinnings and the psychological/behavioral manifestations of alexithymia, thereby improving the effectiveness of our clinical interventions.

The remainder of this paper defines and reviews the concept of alexithymia with a brief description of its neurobiological basis; describes a pilot study of the incidence of alexithymia in a typical neuropsychiatric private practice; discusses standard psychiatric categories in terms of alexithymia; and ends with a glance at the future prospects for a semiotic perspective in neuropsychiatry.

1. Alexithymia: definition and review

Descriptions of alexithymia vary somewhat according to the investigator, clinician or author but there is a general agreement about core features. Although earlier work anticipated his (e.g., Ruesch 1948; MacLean 1949), it was Sifneos (1967, 1973) who in the mid-1960s provided the first conceptualization of alexithymia based on systematic observations of a number of patients suffering from some of the classic psychosomatic illnesses, e.g., peptic ulcer, bronchial asthma. Based on clinical observations, early descriptive efforts characterized the alexithymic as an action oriented (as distinct from relationship or person oriented) individual who suffered from an impoverished fantasy life as well as having great difficulty in identifying feelings. Theoretical efforts focused upon the possibilities that alexithymics were more prone to develop psychosomatic illness as a result of the damming up of feelings, and would be less likely to benefit from the dynamic oriented psychotherapies which required the exploration and articulation of feelings. Sifneos primarily defines alexithymia as a deficiency in the ability to connect emotions with fantasies (Nemiah & Sifneos 1970). The more fully elaborated definition, however, includes four primary distinguishing characteristics.

First, there is a significant difficulty in the identification and description of feelings or a general inability to describe emotions. Descriptions of this characteristic vary according to the author but all note an inconsistency in the use of terms for feelings and emotions. Next, there is an impoverished fantasy life or, as has been otherwise described, a deficiency in symbolic thinking or imaginative abilities. As with the first, descriptions of this deficit remain relatively fuzzy and inconsistent in the literature. The third characteristic pertains to a confusion among feelings, emotions and bodily sensations, sometimes described as an inability to point to various parts of the body where emotions are being felt. Finally, the fourth characteristic refers to an externalizing, operative cognitive style, or a tendency to describe endless and trivial details surrounding an event which was likely to arouse emotions (Bagby, Taylor & Atkinson 1988). This feature incorporates into the description of alexithymia a type of thinking originally labeled by Marty and M'Uzan (1963) as *la pensée opératoire*.

Additional features described by Sifneos include an urgency to act, a tendency to assume rigid postures, diminished capacity to cry or to dream, and deficiencies in experiencing emotions associated with previous events that had been emotionally significant. In spite of variations and inconsistencies in its definition, it is clear that the concept of alexithymia generally represents severe deficiencies in the symbolic and signification processing activities of the individual whereby the identification and appropriate communication of emotions and feelings are compromised.

Originally alexithymia was formulated as an explanatory concept consistent with the notion of "organ neurosis", indicating how blocked or dammed up emotions might result in somatic symptoms. This was the prevailing, largely psychoanalytic, theory behind psychosomatic illnesses, which from the beginning have been imbricated with alexithymia. A second source of interest in alexithymia has come from clinical descriptions of patients who are resistant to or otherwise unable to use psychotherapy as treatment. Marty and M'Uzan, the two French psychiatrists mentioned above (*la pensée opératoire*), described patients who combine both characteristics: they suffer from diverse and nonspecific somatic symptoms and they seldom dream, or cannot report their dreams. These patients' verbalizations are filled with facts and details apparently devoid of emotional significance. Unlike the use of language to create distance in obsessional disorders, these patients' language is described as "present" but *vide* 'empty' (1963). Such patients who are not amenable to talking-type therapies had been described earlier by Ruesch (1948) as "infantile personalities". Ruesch's descriptions are in turn evoked by Sifneos' (1975) and Shands' (1970: 150–171) descriptions of patients who are poor candidates for psychotherapy, and most recently readdressed by Krystal (1979, 1982–1983).

As one of the pioneers in visualizing the usefulness of semiotics for psychiatric practice, Shands clearly saw the symbolic problems of patients who represent illness in one form (soma) that cannot be communicated in another (words). Gradually these clinical descriptions began to focus in on what exactly was not being communicated upon or being miscommunicated both within the individual and between individuals: affects, feelings and emotions. Even as the concept of alexithymia evolves, however, these pieces of the puzzle remain: presence of somatic symptoms and absence of language for emotions. For example, Krystal (1988) takes an up-dated psychoanalytic approach, emphasizing the development of affect regulation, in order to examine alexithymia in relation to traumatic and post-traumatic states and to treatment. Connecting alexithymia with trauma, Krystal raises a currently debated question: namely, are the presence of somatic symptoms and an absence of affect-language due to a stable personality trait of individuals or to a transient, fluctuating or situation-specific coping behavior (e.g., post-traumatic state)? This distinction is sometimes referred to as primary versus secondary alexithymia (Freyberger 1977). (See Ahrens & Deffner 1986 for a review of empirical studies in light of this issue.)

In contrast to clinical descriptions from psychiatric practice, most current research has centered on learning more about this patient population in two ways: by refining measures of identification; and by looking for coexisting psychiatric or physical characteristics. Thus, some studies continue to seek out connections to psychosomatic disorders (e.g., von Rad 1983, 1984; Lolas & von Rad 1989; Keltikangas-Jarvinen 1985, 1987) while others address the incidence of alexithymics among other groups, such as alcohol-dependent or newly abstinent individuals (e.g., Rybakowsky et al. 1988; Haviland et al. 1988; Finn, Martin & Pihl 1987) or depressives (e.g., Haviland et al. 1988). However, determining who is or is not alexithymic has not been a simple task, largely because of unreliable measures.

The earliest measure for alexithymia was a physician administered questionnaire derived directly from Sifneos' research at Beth Israel Hospital in Boston (Beth Israel Questionnaire, BIQ, or Beth Israel Psychosomatic Questionnaire, BIPQ) and supplemented later by two self-reporting measures: the Schalling-Sifneos Personality Scale (SSPS) and the SSPS-Revised. All three scales have 19–20 questions requiring either yes-no or graded answer (A = does not apply at all; B = does not apply very much; C = applies very much; D = applies completely), and all are followed by 12 questions establishing any history of psychosomatic illness (e.g., "Have you ever had: peptic or duodenal ulcer, hypertension, asthma ..."). In addition, alexithymia subscales have been created from the Minnesota Multiphasic Personality Inventory (MMPI). A recent self-reporting measure, the Toronto Alexithymia Scale (TAS), has been found to be superior to others in terms of internal consistency and greater discriminant validity, with a more stable factor structure (Bagby, Taylor & Atkinson 1988). The TAS has 26 questions; graded responses from 1 (strongly disagree) to 5 (strongly agree); and no questions about psychosomatic illnesses. Other measures include varieties of transcript analyses, analyses of responses to projective test stimuli, and another physician administered questionnaire, the Alexithymia Provoked Response Questionnaire (APRQ). (For a description and comparison of these measures see Krystal 1988: chapter 14.)

Although there are many scales now being used to assess alexithymia, some require highly subjective interpretations of responses while others are distinguishing populations on factors which are unclear. For example, analysis of the TAS revealed four factors: ability to describe feelings; ability to identify and distinguish between feelings and bodily sensations; daydreaming; and externally-oriented thinking (Bagby, Taylor & Atkinson 1988: 113). However, using item response theory (Gibbons, Clark & Kupfer n.d.), preliminary analyses of alexithymics responses to the TAS show that only the first two of these, and more specifically a difficulty in finding words for emotions, are really discriminant. What, then, can be said about the relevance to the concept of alexithymia of an inability to daydream/report dreams or the presence of externally-oriented thinking? Although several questions attempt to address these factors, which were part of early clinical descriptions as discussed above, does the TAS adequately measure such features?

Similarly, measures that use projective test stimulus cards, story-telling or other symbolic materials rely on subjective categories of interpretation such as "affect-laden" words, determining "affect magnitude". Responses to these measures have been found to be highly situation and state dependent (Taylor & Doody 1985; Krystal 1988: 296). Some measures assume an underlying symbolic deficit that cuts across all four alexithymic factors (Demers-Desrosiers 1982). Is there such a monolithic symbolic capacity that could go awry, resulting in everything from a misreading of bodily signals to an unimaginative, operative thinking style? Assuming something so global would need to be a part of the brain, several researchers have pursued the concept of alexithymia through split-brain and lateralization studies.

Using measures from transcript analysis (e.g., total words, affect-laden words, specific linguistic categories), some researchers have found a difference in commissuratomized (i.e., split brain) patients versus partially commissuratomized patients, who respond like normal controls (e.g., Hoppe & Bogen 1977). (See studies by Ten Houten et al. 1985a. ,b. ,c.). Such studies assume that emotions processed in the right hemisphere of the brain are isolated from the language processing of the left hemisphere (in right-handed individuals). Using a finger-recognition task, Zeitlin et al. (1989) found differences in the transfer of information between hemispheres in individuals identified as alexithymic and non-alexithymic on the TAS. The trait versus state question arises even in these neurological investigations as some authors have hypothesized a state of "functional commissurotomy" in the face of stress (Ten Houten et al. 1987), i.e., a functional disconnection of the cerebral hemispheres (Buchanan, Waterhouse & West 1980).

These studies pursue an approach that underlay Sifneos' original, neurophysiological conception of alexithymia. The neurophysiology of emotional regulation involves the limbic, autonomic-neuronal, endocrine and neocortical systems. Based on the work of MacLean (1949, 1977) and Hoppe (1977), Sifneos postulated that alexithymia may come about as a result of a breakdown among communication systems within the brain such that the limbic, autonomic, and endocrine systems have no thalamic-neocortical representations which are responsible for conscious awareness of feelings.

Forming a similar conclusion but from a cognitive or information processing approach to emotions (Lazarus 1982; Mandler 1984), Martin et al. (1986) view alexithymia as a result of a "lack of association between physiological and cognitive-behavioral representations within cognitive schemata responsible for mediating affective responses" (1986: 134). Martin & Pihl (1986) measured autonomic responses from frontalis electromyography (FEMG), heart rate (HR) and digital blood volume pulse amplitude (DBVPA) in alexithymic populations. (See also Rabavilas 1987.) These authors report elevated levels of sympathetic activity, i.e., increased levels of arousal, in high alexithymic individuals, but reduced expression and experience of affect. The latter depend upon one's capacity for symbolic cognitive activity, and some authors hypothesize that the various "channels of response" – affective/physiological; cognitive/symbolic; somatic/behavioral – become "decoupled" in alexithymia or were not integrated (e.g., Deffenbacher & Suinn 1982; Vassend 1987; Papciak, Fenerstein & Spiegel 1985). Thus, an inability to communicate to another person about one's affective states may be the result of a deficit in intersystemic communication within the individual. Currently available measures may be too global to specify whence such problems arise in the neurophysiological and cognitive-symbolic systems.

In summary, although we have several means to determine if an individual is or is not alexithymic according to some scale or task, no measure is unequivocal and all are problematic in terms of what they measure. These difficulties directly result from a lack of clarity about the concept of alexithymia, for measures are only instruments derived consciously or unconsciously from one theory or another. Thus, various approaches – psychodynamic, neurological, cognitive – are attempts to provide theoretical models that would explain what goes wrong in alexithymic patients, either in the development of a trait or in a state of transitory regression. Compounding our difficulties is the question of style: an individual's responses may fall within the alexithymic range due to defensive, cognitive, or interactive/communicational styles or may result from socioeconomic status, educational level, gender identification, or other personality traits (Brautigam 1974; von Rad & Lolas 1982; Krystal 1988). (See Lesser 1981, Taylor 1984 and Warnes 1986 for review articles.)

Against this brief review as background I now turn to a description of a pilot study conducted at Rush-Presbyterian-St.Luke's Medical Center, which looks at both diagnosis of alexithymia and its relation to other disorders.

2. Pilot study of alexithymia in a private neuropsychiatric practice

This study sought to compare responses of 32 patients in a typical, neuropsychiatric (private) practice on an accepted measure of alexithymia to their physician's clinical perceptions of the features identified on that measure. The measure used was the TAS because of its superiority to other measures, as noted above. Since this scale was designed to tap key features of alexithymic individuals as clinically described by physicians, the patients' physician in this study was asked to answer questions concerning the presence or absence of these features in his patients.

Thus, the physician was asked the following questions about each patient in the study:

1. Does the patient have a history of somatic illness or a tendency towards somatic reactions?
2. Is the patient now, or has the patient been, chemically dependent; or is the patient now in a state of chemical withdrawal?
3. Has the patient suffered severe trauma, such as parent loss or sexual abuse?
4. Does the patient report frequent dreams or daydreams, and in general have a good imagination with elaborated thoughts?
5. Does the patient know his or her own feelings, and can the patient differentiate and describe feelings?
6. Does the patient prefer things to people and actions to thinking?

The first set of three questions (1 ,2, 3) were meant to assess whether life-historical factors such as somatic illness, trauma or substance abuse, associated with alexithymia in the literature, were known to be factors in these patient's treatment. The second set of three questions (4, 5, 6) were meant to assess whether factors identified as discriminant on the TAS were perceived by these patients' physician as significant. Thus, the TAS scores representing how patients view themselves (since the TAS is a self-report measure) were compared with their physician's perceptions of the same characteristics and with the presence of life-historical factors associated with alexithymia. Each answer was coded 1/0 (yes/no), with responses to negatively-keyed question 6 reversed. A total of 3 points on the first set indicated the highest incidence of life-historical factors, while a total of 3 points on the second set indicated the highest incidence of capacities for representing and expressing emotions, supposedly absent in alexithymics.

Of the thirty-two patients who volunteered to participate in this study 15 were male and 17, female. Their ages ranged from in the 20s to the 50s, distributed as follows: 5 (20–30); 12 (30–40); 12 (40–50); 2 (50+). Data on socioeconomic status and educational level were not collected.

The TAS consists of 26 questions, each of which can be answered by graded responses from 1 to 5, yielding a lowest score of 26 and a highest score of 130. Following Taylor's criteria, scores of 74+ were considered positive for alexithymia; scores of 63– were considered negative for alexithymia; and scores from 64 to 73 are indeterminate. Scores for the patients in this study ranged from 46 to 83, with a mean of 64.15 (S.D. 12.74), distributed as follows: 9 positive (74+); 16 negative (63–); 7 indeterminate (64 to 73). Thus, 28% of this patient population scored within the alexithymic range. Although there were no normal controls in this pilot study, recent studies by Graeme Taylor (personal communication) indicated 18.8% of his normal controls scored within this range. Therefore, it seems reasonable to speculate that a significant number of patients in a typical, private neuropsychiatric practice are alexithymic, according to this measure.

Did those patients who scored within the alexithymic range (74+) present to their physician life-historical factors that have been associated with this condition? No, not every patient with alexithymic scores is perceived by the physician as having a history of those factors. On the other hand, many patients with the highest incidence of life-historical factors (i.e., 3 out of 3 on the first set of questions) also had a score in the high or intermediate alexithymic range. Therefore, while physicians should not expect these factors to automatically signal alexithymia in a patient, a history of somatic illness or tendency towards somatic reactions, chemical dependency and severe trauma should cause a physician to raise the question of possible alexithymia.

A more detailed look at some life-historical factors is revealing. For example, patients who complain of chronic but unspecified pain have scores of 74+, while those who complain of specific pain (e.g., low back pain, headaches) have scores of 63-. Although the numbers of patients in both groups is very small (6 out of 32), these findings are suggestive. All except one patient who scored in the alexithymic range presented a history of somatic illness(es). Similarly, all except one patient who scored in the alexithymic range reported chemical dependency or abuse. While non-alexithymic patients also present with similar histories, complete absence of all three factors (i.e., 0 out of 3 for the first set of questions) occurs in one quarter of the patients and all are not alexithymic on the TAS.

The life-historical factor of trauma was too unspecified to be useful. Furthermore, physicians in a neuropsychiatric practice are not always aware of life traumas suffered by their patients in the past, unless this information has been volunteered by the patient. Interestingly, Krystal who has been the leader in making the connection between alexithymia and trauma, is a psychoanalyst and many of the patients he has studied are holocaust survivors. In contrast, somatic illnesses and symptoms as well as chemical dependency are not only usually volunteered by patients but are often part of their diagnostic categorization in a neuropsychiatric practice. For these reasons, these two factors would seem to be most useful in anticipating a high TAS score. Of these two factors, chemical abuse is the more potent, but especially in combination with nonspecific somatic complaints.

How do patients' responses to questions concerning their abilities to identify feelings, their dreams and imagination, and their preferences for actions over people compare with how their physician perceives these characteristics in them? Comparisons of the physician's responses to the second set of questions had no relationship to TAS scores. For example: it was not the case that 3 points on this set of questions would predict a low TAS score indicative of non-alexithymia; nor was the reverse true. One reason may lie again in the nature of a neuropsychiatric practice: unlike a psychoanalytic practice, this type of information is not usually sought out nor usually volunteered. Another reason may be due to issues raised above in the discussion of measures such as the TAS: it is less sure that in fact they are the best measure of at least two of these factors (dream-imagination and action-people). A third reason may be that truly alexithymic individuals are unreliable respondents to questions concerning their feelings and emotions. Clearly, the use of affect-judgements to assess one's ability to judge affects raises difficult questions about all self-report measures of alexithymia. If in fact some individuals cannot accurately make such judgements, then other self-report measures used in the diagnosis of many psychiatric disorders are equally called into question. As Krystal has noted: "Other self-rating measures in psychiatry may be affected by alexithymic characteristics" and "there is evidence that alexithymia may interfere with psychiatric and medical diagnosis" (1988: 309). For example: The Beck Depression Inventory Rating Scale, widely used in studies of depression, instructs subjects to "circle the correct answer to each question which best describes how you've been feeling over the past week"; a problematic task for an alexithymic who supposedly does not know his feelings and cannot identify emotions or distinguish among them.

The thirty-two patients in this study represented a variety of diagnostic categories. Mention has already been made of somatic symptoms and chemical dependency. In addition, eleven of the thirty-two (34%) were diagnosed as depressed, either alone or in conjunction with other diagnostic categories. Those with diagnoses of depression, major depression, bipolar depression or double depression (6 out of 11) have higher TAS scores (62, 67, 70, 71, 77, 81). In contrast, with one exception those with diagnoses of atypical depression and atypical bipolar depression (5 out of 11) have lower TAS scores (46, 52, 53, 60, 78). The one exception (78) is also the one exception mentioned above in the discussion of chemical dependency: he is the only patient with a positive alexithymia score who did not present with a history of chemical dependency or abuse; he does however have a significant history of somatic illnesses and symptoms. Other researchers have noted the prevalence of alexithymia in patients with diagnosed depressions (see above) and a preliminary study of 16 depressed patients at Rush-Presbyterian-St.Luke's Medical Center shows an incidence rate for alexithymia of 50% (average TAS score of 73.87). Thus, our preliminary data suggest that further investigation of subgroups among different types of depression is warranted.

Besides depression, other psychiatric diagnostic categories have been and should be studied in terms of their relationship to alexithymia. In the treatment research units and in various medical clinics at Rush-Presbyterian-St.Luke's Medical Center we are continuing such studies, as are others elsewhere (e.g., Graeme Taylor in Toronto; Haviland in Loma Linda, California). Current research continues to focus on: the ways that alexithymia may help to differentiate subgroups of a specific disorder such as depression; the development of more precise measures including subscales; and a better understanding of the concept of alexithymia including indepth case studies.

2.1. Implications for semiotics

Both the review of the concept of alexithymia and the review of this pilot research study should be sufficient to indicate the multiple semiotic aspects to alexithymia. In fact, one could argue that alexithymia is a disorder that can only be understood semiotically. And I would further argue that alexithymia is not alone but that in fact all psychiatric diagnostic categories can benefit from a semiotic perspective. Before turning to a discussion of those categories, I would like to make one final comment on the term, *alexithymia*, itself.

Since semiotics is concerned with the meanings of words and with interpretative processes and as these are at issue in any study of the expression of feelings in healthy and pathological conditions, it might be worthwhile to address some problems with the term alexithymia. Based on an expanding literature and empirical observations of a large outpatient and inpatient general psychiatric practice, it appears that alexithymia is relatively ubiquitous, i.e., that it is a spectrum-type disorder, appearing in varying degrees in a wide variety of patients. Furthermore, rarely if ever is there a total or complete incapacity to put one's feelings into words *per se*. Rather, it is a relative incapacity that may represent a state or trait for the individual. Consequently, it would seem more appropriate and accurate to refer to the condition as *dyslexithymia*, 'a disturbed functional capacity for expressing one's feelings in words'. In this regard, it is important to note that this condition in its various forms might relate more to the dyslexias. More might be learned about dyslexithymia by studying the dyslexias than by considering it as an independent condition. A number of the investigations of alexithymia, especially those pertaining to its possible neuroanatomical and neurophysiological features, are suggestive.

3. Categories of psychiatric disorders: DSM-III-R

The fields of semiotics and medicine have been intertwined since antiquity, as many authors have noted. Semiotic considerations are implicit, if not explicit, in the entire spectrum of psychiatric disorders in several ways. First of all, semiotics is implicated in the deceptive nature of symptom formation with respect to the self system and considerations of inner communications at various levels, ranging from somatic through monologic to dialogic. The NATO conference on the semiotics of cellular communication in the immune system exemplifies the usefulness of this perspective at every level (Sercarz, et al. 1988). Similarly, in the interpersonal domain one can look into how intrapersonal and intrapsychic factors contribute to the communicational matrix which so powerfully determine the general patterns and unique features of familial and extra-familial social bondings. Such exploration could profitably be pursued into how defensive operations function to deceive again, with respect to both intrapersonal and interpersonal domains and extending into the social fields. One might even take a look at the cultural representations of these processes and attempt to understand the reflective dynamics whereby they are assimilated back into individual and group lexical dispositions. There is also that special communication between physician and patient wherein symptoms are detected and which is called psychotherapy. But to take a step closer to focusing on the problem of alexithymia let us begin where medicine begins: with diagnosis.

The most basic and comprehensive prevailing model for psychiatry is that proposed by the psychosomatic researcher, George Engel. Some years ago in an article in *Science* (1977), now considered classic, Engel elaborated a bio-psycho-social model. This model is more or less operationalized and codified in terms of a diagnostic classificatory schema, the DSM-III-R, i.e., *Diagnostic and statistical manual of mental disorders* (1987 third edition-revised), developed by the American Psychiatric Association through a concensus building process of committee systems of expert clinicians for the major diagnostic categories.

Both the model and the diagnostic system have been designed to accommodate the inherent complexity of concept, data and description encountered in the scientific study of the interrelationships of behavior and experience. The DSM-III-R which, as an "official" nomenclature, has in addition to its codification significance, far-reaching legal, political, social and economic implications (but these are beyond the scope of this paper). The diagnostic system is multi-axial as follows:

Axis I: contains the major psychiatric, developmental and chemical dependency disorders;
Axis II: contains the personality disorders, many of which are derivative of the neuroses as described in previous terminologies;
Axis III: contains the physical or more purely medical diagnoses;
Axis IV: contains the psychosocial or environmental stressors;
Axis V: contains the highest level of functioning the person achieved during the year prior to diagnosis and is largely behavioral in nature.

A brief clinical vignette might serve as a useful example for understanding research efforts designed to investigate the alexithymic phenomenon more broadly and in greater depth. A typical patient who suffers from alexithymia is likely to have a treatment refractory psychiatric disorder such as a major depression or generalized anxiety disorder with panic attacks as a DSM-III-R Axis I diagnosis. Somatic features such as headaches, myalgia and/or gastrointestinal problems such as spastic colon are likely. An Axis II diagnosis of a mixed or specific personality disorder such as passive-dependency would not be unusual. On Axis III, the patient might indeed suffer from a peptic ulcer, mitral valve prolapse or neurodermatitis. In addition, it would not be unusual for the patient to have had one or more courses of unsuccessful psychotherapy or pharmacotherapy; and the patient is very likely to be using excessive amounts of alcohol and/or prescription drugs to self-medicate in an attempt to relieve both the somatic distress and painful affect states that are poorly identified and not expressed.

What is interesting about DSM-III-R with respect to my topic is that although so many of the diagnoses referred to are based upon disorders of affect or emotion, there is virtually no reference to a phenomenon ubiquitous in clinical psychiatric practice, i.e., that of alexithymia or the relative inability of a person to give verbal expression to their feelings. Indeed, a major, if not "the", goal of so much of psychotherapeutic (and by extension, pharmacotherapeutic) endeavors is to facilitate or enable the persons being treated to get "in touch" with their feelings, i.e., to be able to find the appropriate means of emotional expression. The key therapeutic significance of alexithymia is emphasized by Krystal who states that it "is the single most important cause of poor outcome or outright failure of psychoanalysis and psychoanalytic psychotherapy" (1988: xi). More generally, the effectiveness of psychotherapy is based upon a multiplicity of factors associated with the dyadic interactional processing of emotionally significant verbal material while that of psychopharmacotherapy relies upon the neurochemical modulation of signaling processes within neurophysiological substrata, serving emotional behavior. In both circumstances, the relative ability of the patient to identify and discuss feelings reflect critical symbolic processing features of their self system and is of prime significance to the therapist responsible for the direction and specification of treatment.

Not that the DSM-III-R ignores these issues. Affect is defined as "a pattern of observable behaviors that is the expression of a subjectively experienced feeling state (emotion)" (1987: 391). Affect, "variable over time", is differentiated from mood, "a pervasive and sustained emotion" (1987: 401). Some patients are described as using "empty speech" but it is not clear how such poverty of content should be measured. Psychosomatic pathologies are described under somatoform disorders (1987: 255), including hypochondriasis, hysteria, atypical somatoform disorder, psychogenic pain disorder, and conversion disorder. The last is "unique in this classification" because the "symptom has symbolic value that is a representation and partial solution of the underlying psychological conflict" (1987: 257). These disorders were described by Freud in his classic studies of conversion hysteria. The DSM-III-R, however, does not differentiate symptoms that have symbolic value from those that do not; and symptoms are considered equivalent to signs (1987: 405); i.e., not a particular kind of sign.

3.1. Prospects for a semiotic perspective in neuropsychiatry

This paper has been concerned with the clinical significance and theoretical implications that result from approaching the concept of alexithymia from a semiotic perspective. Since the essential deficits associated with alexithymia appear to be most cogently conceptualized in terms of symbolic and signification processing disturbances with respect to the emotions in general, it seems most appropriate to utilize the perspective of contemporary clinical semiotics to explore the clinical and theoretical ramifications of alexithymia. Although this approach of employing a contemporary semiotic perspective represents an original theoretical exploration and scientific investigation into a clinical subject of increasing current interest and significance, as noted above the intertwining of medicine and semiotics is not a new pursuit. This current effort to meaningfully integrate these scientific and philosophic-humanistic disciplines has, in addition to enhancing our understanding of alexithymia and extending the parameters of applied semiotics, the potential consequence of practical therapeutic advances for those who may suffer from a wide variety of neuropsychiatric disorders, especially for those in whom alexithymia is involved. I have tried to show that this involvement may cut across all neuropsychiatric diagnostic categories. In addition, hopefully this exposition will serve as a step in the development of a model of clinical semiotics that will help to elucidate a clinical lexicon and to generate a scientific discourse that addresses the needs of clinicians, researchers, and theoreticians by creating a common language that can coordinate, integrate and unify knowledge among the various disciplines concerned with the neuropsychological and sociocultural sciences and health professionals. Semiotics, strongly rooted in philosophy, discourse, linguistics, social and cultural anthropology and related systems of thought provides a theoretical perspective and methodological advantages that promise to make important inroads to the study of alexithymia and related clinical problems.

Consequently, I foresee two major types of contributions that could result from a semiotic perspective: the first having to do with an understanding of the expression of emotions and the ways in which this figures into various psychopathological states; the second having to do with a common vocabulary that would enable constructive interdisciplinary discourse. In his *Project for a scientific psychology* (1895), as well as in other works, Freud elaborated on the "signal" theory of anxiety as it pertains to defensive and regulatory operations with respect to primary and secondary process mental functioning. Since the very nature of the associative process in normal and psychopathological conditions depends on a system of signaling processes, clearly semiotic theory and methods can provide a theoretical framework (consistent with other social and communicational sciences) to investigate how signals basic to neuroscience become elaborated into the symbols and signs of human-environmental interactions.

Apart from the natural phenomena themselves, i.e., the functioning of the central nervous system as it pertains to the regulation and expression of moods, feelings, and emotions in their myriad forms, the language forms we use to codify the information and knowledge that we generate and rely upon to provide the structure of our understanding (for example, the DSM-III-R) is problematic itself. Concurrent with our empirical investigations into the nature of the clinical phenomena we wish to understand better, we must closely scrutinize our own use of language in the generation of concepts used to organize information and ideas into knowledge worthy of the designation of science. And this is especially important when we are concerned with the science of mind and the topic of emotion. In a general sense, then, we are concerned with the features and qualities of scientific discourse even as we are engaged in that discourse. To be unaware of the constraints and problems associated with the language forms we use, especially in clinical neuropsychiatric endeavors is to be guilty of ignoring confounding variables of the most persistent type that contribute to ongoing distortions of "scientific reality", that obfuscate at best and generate hypocrisy and theoretical fraud at worst. Herein lies the basis and justification for employing a semiotic perspective from which to view both the phenomena in question and the discourse about the phenomena.

Riordan has compared a scientific community in its relentless pursuit of objective truth to a "vast collective mind" (1987: 369). Of paramount importance to growth is the free and rapid exchange of information among its many parts; and at the heart of this exchange sits language. So the truth scientists speak about is not some rigid, static entity "out there", but a living, growing, evolving body of successful ideas shared with colleagues. From psychoanalysis we can draw the concept of the "observing ego" which functions as a key psychological instrument for the development of insight which in turn provides one with introspective abilities to reflect upon one's feelings, thoughts and actions with increased objectivity. I am suggesting that the formal application of semiotics to science in general and especially to our systematic attempts to understand mind, behavior and emotion (and their interrelationships) will serve the function of providing an observing eye for the collective mind of science.

In this chapter my goal has been to lay the groundwork for the establishment of the theoretical rationale and initial steps for the introduction of semiotics into empirical clinical investigations of a specific dysfunction, alexithymia. Involving as it does both neurophysiologic and symbolic functioning, alexithymia provides an ideal opportunity to demonstrate the usefulness of a semiotic approach to neuropsychiatry.

References

Ahrens, Stephen & Gerhard Deffner
1986 "Empirical study of alexithymia: methodology and results", American-*Journal of Psychotherapy* 40 no. 3, 430–447.

Bagby, R. Michael , Graeme J. Taylor & Leslie Atkinson
1988 "Alexithymia: a comparative study of three self-report measures", *Journal of Psychosomatic Research* 32, 107–116.

Brautigam, Walter
1974 "Pathogenetische Therapien und Wege der Behandlung in der Psychosomatik", *Nervenarzt* 45, 354–363.

Buchanan, Denton C., Gloria J. Waterhouse & Sam C. West
1980 "A proposed neurophysiological basis of alexithymia", *Psychotherapy and Psychosomatics* 34, 248–255.

Cheren, Stanley (ed.)
1989 *Psychosomatic medicine: theory, physiology and practice.* Vol. 1. New York: International Universities Press.

Deffenbacher, Jerry L. & Richard M. Suinn
1982 "The self-control of anxiety", in: Paul Karoly & Frederick Kanfer (eds.), 393–443.

Demers-Desrosiers, Louise A.
1982 "Influence of alexithymia on symbolic function", *Psychotherapy and Psychosomatics* 38, 103–120.

Diagnostic and statistical manual of mental disorders. (3rd edition-revised.)
1987 Washington DC: American Psychiatric Association, 1987.

Engel, George
1977 "The need for a new medical model: a challenge for biomedicine", *Science* 196 (4286), 129–136.

Finn, Peter R., John B. Martin & Robert O. Pihl
1987 "Alexithymia in males at high genetic risk for alcoholism", *Psychotherapy and Psychosomatics* 47, 18–21.

Freud, Sigmund
1895 *Project for a scientific psychology.* S.E. I, 281–397. London: The Hogarth Press.

Freyberger, Hellmuth
1977 "Supportive psychoterapeutic techniques in primary and secondary alexithymia", *Psychotherapy and Psychosomatics* 2, 337–342.
Gibbons, Robert D., David C. Clark & David J. Kupfer
n.d. "Full information item factor analysis of the Hamilton Depression Rating Scale". [Unpublished manuscript.]
Haviland, Mark G., Dale G. Shaw, Michael A. Cummings & James P. MacMurray
1988 "Subscales and relationship to depression", *Psychotherapy and Psychosomatics* 50: 164–170.
Haviland, Mark G., Dale G. Shaw, James P. MacMurray & Michael A. Cummings
1988 "Validation of the Toronto Alexithymia Scale with substance abusers", *Psychotherapy and Psychosomatics* 50, 81–87.
Hill, Oscar (ed.)
1970 *Modern trends in psychosomatic medicine*. Vol. 2. London: Butterworth
Hoppe, Klaus D.
1977 "Split brain and psychoanalysis", *Psychoanalytic Quarterly* 46, 22–244.
Hoppe, Klaus D. & Joseph E. Bogen
1977 "Alexithymia in twelve commisurotomized patients", *Psychotherapy and Psychosomatics* 28, 148–155.
Karoly, Paul & Frederick Kanger (eds.)
1982 *Self-management and behavior change: from theory to practice*. New York: Pergamon.
Keltikangas-Järvinen, Liisa
1985 "Concept of alexithymia I: prevalence of alexithymia in psychosomatic patients", *Psychotherapy and Psychosomatics* 44, 132–138.
1987 "Concept of alexithymia II: the consistency of alexithymia", *Psychotherapy and Psychosomatics* 47, 113–120.
Krystal, Henry
1979 "Alexithymia and psychotherapy", *American Journal of Psychotherapy* 33, 17–28.
1982 "Alexithymia and the effectiveness of psychoanalytic treatment", International Journal of Psychoanalytic Psychotherapy 9, 353–388.
1988 *Integration and self-healing: affect-trauma-alexithymia*. Hillsdale, NJ: The Analytic Press.
Lazarus, Richard S.
1982 "Thoughts on the relations between emotion and cognition", *American Psychologist* 37, 1019–1024.
Lesser, Ira
1981 "A review of the alexithymia concept", *Psychosomatic Medicine* 43, 531–543.

Lolas, Fernando & Michael von Rad
1989 "Alexithymia", in: S. Cheren (ed.), 189-237.
MacLean, Paul D.
1949 "Psychosomatic disease and the 'visceral brain'", *Psychosomatic Medicine* 11, 338-353.
1977 "The triune brain in conflict", *Psychotherapy and Psychosomatics* 28, 207–220.
Mandler, George
1984 *Mind and body: psychology emotion and stress*. New York: Norton.
Martin, John B. & Robert O. Pihl
1986 "Influence of alexithymic characteristics on physiological and subjective stress responses in normal individuals", *Psychotherapy and Psychosomatics* 45, 66–77.
Martin, John B., Robert O. Pihl, Simon N. Young, Frank R. Ervin & Smadar V. Tourjman
1986 "Prediction of alexithymic characteristics from physiological, personality, and subjective measures", *Psychotherapy and Psychosomatics* 45, 133–140.
Marty, Pierre & Michel de M'Uzan
1963 "La pensée opératoire", *Revue Française Psychanalyse* 27. suppl., 345–356.
Nemiah, John & Peter Sifneos
1970 "Affect and fantasy in patients with psychosomatic disorders", in: Oscar Hill (ed.), 26–34.
Papciak, Anthony S., Michael Fenerstein & Jodi A. Spiegel
1985 "Stress reactivity in alexithymia: decoupling of physiological and cognitive responses", *Journal of Human Stress* 11, 135–142.
Rabavilas, Andreas D.
1987 "Electrodermal activity in low and high alexithymia neurotic patients", *Psychotherapy and Psychosomatics* 47, 101–104.
Rad, Michael von (ed.)
1983 *Alexithymie - empirische Untersuchungen zur Diagnostik und Therapie psychosomatisch Kranker*. Berlin: Springer Verlag.
Rad, Michael von
1984 "Alexithymia and symptom formation", *Psychotherapy and Psychosomatics* 42, 80–89.
Rad, Michael von & Fernando Lolas
1982 "Empirical evidence of alexithymia", *Psychotherapy and Psychosomatics* 38, 91–102.

Riordan, Michael
1987 *The hunting of the quark: a true story of modern physics*. New York Simon & Schuster/Touchstone.
Ruesch, Jürgen
1948 "The infantile personality as the core problem of psychosomatic medicine", *Psychosomatic Medicine* 10, 134–142.
Rybakowski, Janusz, Marcin Ziolkowski, Teresa Zasadska & Roman Brzezinski
1988 "High prevalence of alexithymia in male patients with alcohol dependence", *Drug and Alcohol Dependence* 21, 133–136.
Sercarz, E.E., F. Celada, N.A. Mitchison & T. Tada (eds.)
1988 *The semiotics of cellular communication in the immune system*. Berlin: Springer-Verlag.
Shands, Harley
1970 *Semiotic approaches to psychiatry*. The Hague: Mouton.
Sifneos, Peter
1967 "Clinical observations on some patients suffering from a variety of psychosomatic diseases", *Acta medica psychosomatica*. Proceedings of the 7th European Conference on Psychosomatic Research, Rome, September 11–16, 452–458.
1973 "The prevalence of 'alexithymic' characteristics in psychosomatic patients", *Psychotherapy and Psychosomatics* 22, 255–262.
1975 "Problems of psychotherapy of patients with alexithymic characteristics and physical disease", *Psychotherapy and Psychsomatics* 26, 65–70.
Taylor, Graeme J.
1984 "Alexithymia: concept, measurement and implications for treatment", *American Journal of Psychiatry* 141, 725–732.
Taylor, Graeme J. & Kenneth Doody
1985 "Verbal measures of alexithymia: what do they measure", *Psychotherapy and Psychosomatics* 43, 32–37.
Ten Houten, W.D., Klaus D. Hoppe, Joseph E. Bogen & D.O. Walter
1985a "Alexithymia and the split brain II: sentential-level content analysis", *Psychotherapy and Psychosomatics* 44, 1–5.
1985b "Alexithymia and the split brain III: global level content analysis of fantasy and symbolization", *Psychotherapy and Psychosomatics* 44, 89–94.
1985c "Alexithymia and the split brain IV: Gottschalk-Glesser content analysis, an overview", *Psychotherapy and Psychosomatics* 44, 113–121.
Vassend, Olav
1987 "Personality, imaginative involvement and self-reported somatic complaints: relevance to the concept of alexithymia", *Psychotherapy and Psychosomatics* 47, 74–81.

Warnes, H.
1986 "Alexithymia, clinical and therapeutic aspects", *Psychotherapy and Psychosomatics* 46, 91–104.
Zeitlin, Sharon, Richard Lane, Daniel O'Leary & Michael Schrift
1989 "Interhemispheric transfer deficit and alexithymia", *American Journal of Psychiatry* 146 no. 11, 1434–1439.

Pharmacosemiotics: where is the message in the drug?

F. Eugene Yates

Therapeutic drugs are molecular agents of a physician's purpose. The physician intends to make the patient better by introducing a carefully selected chemical species into the complex system that is the human subject, with the expectation that a causal sequence of events will be initiated, leading to macroscopic changes observed by the physician, or felt by the patient. If the patient is hypertensive, the drug lowers the blood pressure and this is a physical change observable by the physician. Usually, the patient does not feel this change. At the other extreme, if a patient is having an acute anginal attack (i.e., heart pain in the chest), a sublingual tablet of nitroglycerin may quickly relieve the pain and anxiety, without objective signs detectable by the physician. (There may be electrocardiographic changes that the physician could detect.) In either case, whether the end point of the therapy is an objectively observed or subjectively felt change in state of the patient, we try to give a causal rationale for the therapy. For example, if the blood pressure lowering drug is a member of the class of so-called "calcium entry blockers" such as verapamil, nifedipine, or diltiazem, we say that the drug caused vasodilation of the arteriolar resistance vessels by reducing the "tone" of the smooth muscle in their walls by changing the availability of ionized calcium. Similarly, mechanistic accounts are used to describe the anti-anginal effects of nitroglycerin: we imagine that the drug decreases the "preload" on the heart, and therefore its oxygen requirement, by relaxing the smooth muscles of large veins, thereby reducing central venous pressure and the filling of the heart during diastole.

It is a considerable triumph of modern pharmaceutical research, based whenever possible on molecular and cell biology, as well as on whole animal and clinical testing, that we are able to tell a causal story for most drug therapies. These stories do not suggest the need for any kind of meta-analysis or semiotic perspective. Unfortunately, our simple, Newtonian-causal views are inadequate to account for some peculiar aspects of drug therapy. We must go beyond the Newtonian view to understand these peculiarities. But first, it is useful to reflect on the deep influence that the Newtonian picture of the world has had on scientific thinking in all fields, including pharmaceutical sciences.

1. Newtonian causality

Robert Rosen has explored the concept of causality in physics and biology in a series of four very deep and thoughtful papers (1986). In this section I paraphrase his ideas.

The Newtonian system of mechanics provided a universal procedure for dealing with material phenomena consisting of particles and forces. The paradigm he offered has become the basis of modern system theory, but goes farther than that: it pervades almost all reductionistic science. The Newtonian paradigm is deeply causal: it supposes that all you need to know is a present state plus a dynamical law to determine the next state and all subsequent states. Here let me emphasize that the notion of cause is not an essential part of physics, and is in fact often deplored by physicists, just as the notion of purpose in biology makes modern biologists uneasy. Nevertheless, both concepts seem intuitively needed for satisfying, if not satisfactory, explanations. The strong appeal of the Newtonian paradigm was that it provided a view from which every system could be seen as simple in prin-ciple. Nevertheless, the specific Newtonian algorithm for analysis of material systems has failed very badly in biology because it does not account for things like organisms. The properties of organisms, particularly turnover of materials, growth and development, have been very difficult to integrate into the Newtonian world view. Even before Newton, and on to the present day, the inventors of physics have sought universal laws applicable to all of material nature. Living systems seemed always too special to suggest biology as an area in which universal laws might be found. Organisms are nongeneric; their richness lies in the many initial conditions, boundary conditions, and constraints which must be independently specified in order to bring the universals of physics to bear upon them. Physics is about simple systems; organisms are complex.

2. Complexity

According to Rosen, the essence of complexity is that an organism can present itself to different observers in a way that can be described simply (that is, according to the standard Newtonian paradigm), but the simple description will be different for different observers. A complex system cannot be comprehensibly described as a whole; it admits a multiplicity of partial descriptions. According to this view, complexity is not an intrinsic property of systems, but depends on the modes of interaction with (e.g., observation of) the system available to us. If we can interact with a system in only a few ways, it will appear simple to us. An organism is complex because we can interact with it in many ways, no one of which suffices to characterize it. Furthermore, the complex system itself is not in any sense a superposition of the simple, partial descriptions. This departure from superposition, which is a technical and basic analytical feature of the study of simple physical systems, is even taken occasionally to be a definition of complexity. Departure from superposition defeats any attempt to generate a comprehensive account of an organism through methodological reduction to mechanism or syntax. (See Ayala 1987 for an account of varieties of reductionism in modern science.)

3. Syntactics as scientific reductionism

Syntax was originally a linguistic concept pertaining to patterns of arrangement of lexical units. It emphasized that which was true in a language solely because of form and pattern, independent of any other considerations. By avoiding study of meaning or signification (i.e., semantics), syntax appears objective and "scientific", free of the subjectivities of semantics that entail polysemes and ambiguities. The power of the syntactical reduction in science is seen in the mathematical process called formalization. As described by Kleene (1952: 7):

> This step (formalization) will not be finished until all the properties of the undefined or technical terms of the theory which matter for the deduction of theorems have been expressed by axioms. It should then be possible to perform the deductions by treating the technical terms as words in themselves without meaning – for to say that they have meanings necessary to the deductions of the theorems, other than what they derive from the axioms which govern them, amounts to saying that not all of their properties which matter for the deductions have been expressed by axioms. When the meanings of the technical terms are thus left out of account, we have arrived at the standpoint of formal axiomatics ... Since we have abstracted entirely from the content matter, leaving only the form, we say that the original theory has been formalized. In this structure, the theory is no longer a system of meaningful propositions, but one of sentences as sequences of words, which are in turn sequences of letters. We say by reference to the form alone which combinations of words are sentences, which sentences are axioms, and which sentences follow as immediate consequences from others.

Kleene obviously thought that any system could be formalized and that formalization itself, which is a purely syntactic entity devoid of any meaning, is fully equivalent to the original system which it formalizes. In his view, formalization loses no information present in the original system; it is only a reformulation. Axioms generate theorems by syntactic production rules. The field of Artificial Intelligence can be seen as a current manifestation of the trend toward pure syntactics that has grown up in mathematics, logic and physics in the Newtonian paradigm. There is a strong similarity between mathematics as the manipulation of meaningless, unanalyzable symbols according to fixed syntactic rules and physical systems as collections of elementary units manipulated by definite forces, represented by dynamical laws or rules. The core of the reductionistic program in all sciences is the belief that every mathematical truth can be generated in purely syntactic terms or, similarly, the belief that every physical truth translates into a truth about atoms and forces.

With the above heuristic arguments as background, I turn now to an example of a spectacular failure of the Newtonian paradigm and syntactical approach in pharmacology.

4. Set and setting

In 1972 Andrew Weil published a popular book arising out of his interest in "thinking about drugs and consciousness". Early in the book he remarks on a phenomenon well known in pharmacology, but not greatly emphasized: the importance of set and setting in determining a person's reaction to a psychoactive drug:

> During the year that our drug ring operated out of Claverly Hall, I had a chance to watch perhaps 30 mescaline experiences of other undergraduates, and, again, what was most striking was the variability of these sessions. All the experiences were mostly pleasant, with no bad reactions, but no two were alike, even in the same person. What we were seeing was also being noted by (Timothy) Leary and (Richard) Alpert in their continuing studies with psilocybin. They gave the drug to large numbers of intellectuals, artists, alcoholics, prisoners, addicts, and graduate students; reported that the vast majority of the experiences were positive; and pointed out the importance of "set" and "setting" in determining the subject's reaction. Set is a person's expectations of what a drug will do to him, considered in the context of his whole personality. Setting is the environment, both physical and social, in which a drug is taken. Leary and Alpert were the first investigators of the hallucinogens to insist on the importance of these two variables. Without them, we are unable to explain simply why the drug varies so unpredictably in its psychic effects from person to person and from time to time in the same person. With these variables, the observations become suddenly clear; hence the usefulness of the concept of set and setting (1972: 29).

As is well known, Harvard University dismissed Richard Alpert and Timothy Leary in 1963. Their investigations, and the book by Weil, consisted of anecdotes not taken seriously as scientific evidence. Nevertheless, the concepts of set and setting as establishing a context that influences the (apparent) action of a drug remain fundamental for the understanding of psychotropic agents. The principles are generalizable and can be captured in the phrase: context is the operator! In the case of drugs or drug actions not involving the brain, context may be entirely an internal matter and may be synonymous with physiological state, but because of the high number of internal degrees of freedom in biochemical networks, internal state can never be precisely specified and is always only partially known. Therefore, I view a high-dimensional state as providing a context that operates to shape the dynamic changes intended by the physician when he administers a drug. These dynamic changes are, loosely, an interpretation of a message provided by the drug therapy. I realize that, by introducing the word "message" in a sentence about dynamics, I am obligated to offer some kind of bridge between the world of dynamics (e.g., state transitions) and that of information.

5. Information versus dynamics in living systems

Dynamics is about motion and change, whereas information is static, not dependent upon or involving rates. Howard Pattee views information and dynamics as being complementary aspects of complex systems (Pattee 1977, 1978, 1982, 1985, 1987). The two concepts intersect in our notions that information as static structure constrains and specifies dynamics, and that a flow of information (implying rates) can command a dynamic system to change its state. Elsewhere I have described these concepts and their applicability to living systems in greater detail (Yates 1982, 1985, 1988; Yates & Kugler 1984). More specifically, I have suggested that molecular receptors act as a bridge between information and dynamics in living systems (Yates 1987). There I remarked:

> The convergence of biology and physics, if it ever occurs, will result, I believe, from rationalization of information using terms and concepts of physics. At the moment it does not seem profitable to attempt that demonstration in the fields of neurosciences, immunology or genetics because these branches of biology are too thoroughly permeated with the information metaphor. A better opportunity lies in the analysis of receptors. Receptors bind chemicals in their environment (the "recognition" step) and modulate dynamic contingencies or actions within the cells bearing the receptors, the "activation" step. Activation usually involves chemical cas-

> cades as amplifiers, and mappings from variations of one chemical species into those of another, the "second messenger". Second messengers in the chain of events centered on the receptor are very often fluxes of calcium ions or cyc-lic nucleotides ... Whatever the mechanistic details, receptors stand between environmental, chemical variations and those cellular dynamic changes that biologists informally regard as "interpretations" of the environment. In the field of receptor biology the techniques of quantum chemistry, chemical kin-etics, cell physiology and gene-cloning-probes intersect. It is here, if any-where, that information emerges from dynamics (1987: 633).

6. Receptors

We are indebted to Paul Ehrlich (1913) and J. N. Langley (1909) for providing experimental data and theoretical constructs that have led to the modern concept of drug-receptor interaction as a basis of chemotherapeutics. Ehrlich had noticed the high degree of antibody specificity against antigenic substances and he imagined a stereospecific lock-and-key fit between them. Later, in his work on chemotherapy involving interactions between synthetic organic chemicals and parasitic protozoa, he again observed a high degree of specificity. Small variations in a drug's chemical structure affected both its therapeutic potency and its toxicity. Ehrlich imagined that the protoplasm of cells presented chemical side chains (that he called receptors) to its outside environment, on which chemotherapeutic substances had to act. He went so far as to introduce the rule that drugs cannot act unless they are bound to receptors, though today we know of some exceptions.

John Newport Langley came to similar conclusions from a different line of evidence. He found that the South American arrow poison, curare, could stop transmission of impulses from motor nerves to skeletal muscles. When motor nerves were cut and allowed to degenerate, the muscle cells could still be stimulated chemically, as by nicotine. Curare could stop that action of nicotine as well as it had stopped the action of nerve stimulation on the muscle. Yet even during curare blockade, either in innervated or denervated muscle, direct electrical stimulation of the muscle would still cause contraction. He concluded that nicotine and curare must act on some substance that is neither nerve nor muscle! He referred to this as the "receptive substance". We now know it as the acetylcholine receptor of the motor endplate, and take the view that most drug actions occur through receptor recognition-activation, amplifying processes. The effects of drug-receptor interaction ultimately are changes in ongoing dynamics or dynamic contingencies of cells (Goldstein, Aronow & Kalman 1974). The conventional, reductionistic approach to the study of ligand-receptor interaction can be found in the new book by

Darnell, Lodish and Baltimore (1986). The chief ideas are that: (1) hydrophilic molecules act by binding to cell surface receptors; (2) small lipophilic molecules diffuse through the plasma membrane and interact with cytosolic or nuclear receptors; and (3) large lipophilic molecules bind to plasma membrane receptors.

Binding of a ligand to cell surface receptors triggers an increase or decrease in the cytosolic concentration of cyclic adenosine monophosphate (cAMP), calcium ion (Ca2+), or some other "second messenger" substance. Other ligands that bind interiorly, to specific receptors in the cytosol or nucleus, act more directly on nuclear deoxyribonucleic acid (DNA) to increase transcription of specific genes. In this scheme, all the information in a physician's therapeutic command lies in the structure of the drug (ligand). But the scheme is impoverished because it leads to the impression, contrary to fact, that the same drug at the same concentration would lead to the same effect on the same cells whenever it was bound to their receptors.

To the above reductionistic scheme, based on the root metaphor of the machine (Pepper 1942), we must add a dose of contextualism, with the root metaphor of the historical event or acts in a context. The context arises from the uniqueness of the genome of the receiving cell, from the chemical field in which the cell is embedded (including other signals at other receptors), the recent past (cells have nonlinear processes acting as "memories"), the amplitude of the signal (the thermodynamic activity of the ligand drug – i.e., approximately its concentration in the fluid outside the cell) and, finally, variations in thermodynamic activity in time – the pattern of concentration over time (including amplitude modulation of the signal, frequency modulation, and/or rate-sensitivity). In the history of psychology, contextualism has a recognized place (Lerner, Hultsch and Dixon 1983). For example, Lewin (1935) drew a contrast between what he called Aristotelian and Galilean modes of thought. Lewin noted that causality can be understood either from a "cross-sectional" perspective or from a "longitudinal" perspective. He called the longitudinal causality Aristotelian or historical (i.e., contextual), and the cross-sectional causality Galilean or ahistorical (I would say, Newtonian). In this dichotomization Aristotelian causality considers such factors as genetic contributions to longitudinal, individual personality development; Galilean causality considers instead all of the field forces currently acting on the person that will influence his behavior. I now suggest that these same issues debated in developmental psychology can be found at the endosemiotic level of drug action: the field I call *pharmacosemiotics*.

It may be objected, of course, that by introducing pharmacosemiotics I am dealing in archaic tropes and metaphors rather than in modern truth and mechanism. My reply is that the influences of set and setting, the recognized drug interactions, the phenomenon of drug tolerance, the problems of drug idiosyncracy, allergy and resistance – all imply that drug effects are multicausal. They force us to consider context as an operator in pharmacology. Just as the word *bear* can be given two readings and two meanings, depending on context, the structure of a drug, playing the role of the structure of a word, requires context for its interpretation and signification. One aspect of the context is self-referential; namely, its own concentration! As the dose of a drug is increased, we may see not just progressively stronger responses of the same kind, but new responses sometimes reversing a preceding response (e.g., bradycardia changing to tachycardia; many anesthetic agents excite at low doses and depress at higher doses). In addition, some drugs that are antagonists also have intrinsic agonist activity. For example, pindolol is a synthetic beta-adrenergic receptor blocking agent with intrinsic sympathomimetic activity mediated directly at the adrenergic receptor sites and blockable by other beta-blockers.

7. Beyond structure-activity relationships

Conventional pharmacology supposes that with respect to a biologically active agent, the chemical properties determine its action and activity. A relationship exists between structure and action, although it is not always readily recognized (Ariens 1979). I have objected to this view on the grounds that it is too limited (Yates 1979). I pointed out that although there is necessarily a structural, chemical complementarity between a receptor and a ligand for the process of recognition, there is no such obligatory relationship between a ligand structure and subsequent cellular activation. The structure of a drug molecule has little or no bearing on its cellular interpretation. The molecule is not the message; it is a morpheme in a language whose syntactical rules are executed by structures to generate dynamical interpretations according to a context. In drug therapy, meaning depends upon lexical units, their ordering according to syntax, and context as an operator to shape interpretations and assign significance. That the context is provided by chemical fields rather than by acoustic phenomena (hearing) or photon fluxes (seeing) does not vitiate the argument that the underlying phenomena belong in the domain of semiotic inquiry. Chemical fields influence transports and transformations of matter and energy micro-tactilely (by touch).

8. Molecular semiosis

Peirce decreed that semiosis, or the interpretation of signs, can know no end. A concern of proponents of limitless semiosis is how easily one might lose touch with reality under the sheer mass of meaningfulness in the world. Committed semioticians may be better off to live switched off for a good part of the time lest they become submerged by the impossible richness of meaning in everything they see and hear. The lure of excessive meaningfulness is a semiotic thread that Umberto Eco has woven through his novels. Or, as Thomas Wolfe wrote: Man looks to the indifferent stars and assigns his own meanings. His genes, life experiences and present circumstances provide the operative context. Is it the same at the molecular level, with cells?

Gordon Tomkins (1975) was one of the first biochemists to recognize that chemical potentials in a chemical field act as signs and symbols to receptive cells. He even suggested the term "metabolic code", in contrast to genetic code, to indicate that chemical fields have significance to cells which they can interpret broadly as, for example, hunger. Having made that interpretation, they can alter their behavior in a beneficial way; either to search for and find the missing nutrient, or by erecting defenses against the shortage. Having interpreted the symbol, they make a decision. Semiosis begins with cells. I agree fully with Sebeok who remarked with respect to the work of the biologist Lynn Margulis:

> I think it is better to talk about cells as the first pieces of machinery that process signs ... Signs, or semiosis, I reserve for the time that cells appeared. The amazing thing that happened after that is that between the appearance of the first cell, again roughly 4 billion years ago, for an enormously long time ... the only things that were alive were tiny, single-cell organisms we call prokaryotes ... The life of these prokaryotes is quite remarkable ... Many of these prokaryotic microorganisms form specific relationships that are called, in biological jargon, symbiosis. Symbiosis means that two or more organisms live cooperatively in such a way that each depends on the other in some crucial way for its subsistence, or even its long-term survival. I submit that the words symbiosis that biologists use is nothing but a form of semiosis, that is to say, these organisms exchange signs, and eventually the sign exchanges among them become so complicated that a new mechanism evolves ... (1987: 13–14).

A consequence, I believe, of the semiotic nature of biological molecular processes is that cells use very functional commands. They can read or parse a chemical field, picking out of its complexion a symbol interpreted as impending starvation, and then act on that interpretation by making a decision to aggregate with other cells, as the free-swimming amoebae of the slime mold do under such circumstances (see the accounts by Garfinkel 1987 and Tomkins 1975). As another example, consider the multiple factors required for growth, as opposed to mere survival of the culture, in chemically defined cell culture media; they seem to be mostly mitogenic triggers that appear to say: Divide!

In pharmacosemiotics the emphasis is on sequence, phase, wave forms or order of events as the independent variables, rather than more conventionally on time or on plasma concentrations in the steady state. There are at least five aspects of concentration wave forms that might possess "information" (Yates & Poston 1986). These are: (1) level or static dose-response; (2) frequency of an oscillation; (3) phase of an oscillation; (4) threshold for switching; and (5) rate-of-change of level or frequency. Of these five items, only item (1) is traditionally treated in pharmacology. For example, in chapter 2, "Pharmacodynamics: mechanisms of drug action and the relationship between drug concentration and effect", by Ross and Gilman, of the now classic Goodman and Gilman's *The pharmacological basis of therapeutics* (Gilman, et al. 1985), only steady-state mass or concentration amplitudes appear as independent variables provoking therapeutic effects. The more dynamic aspects of oscillatory or rate-sensitive properties are not addressed, even though over 25 years ago Clynes (1961, 1962) showed the importance of unidirectional rate sensitivity as a basis of some nonlinear properties of humeral systems; and for the same length of time Halberg (1969) has repeatedly demonstrated the importance of oscillatory phase and amplitude in physiology and chemotherapy. The reason for the neglect of these higher-order aspects of concentration wave forms of chemicals in biological fluids as sources of "information" or "meaning" is easy to find: they are difficult to deal with experimentally and there is no obvious way to prepare a biological system for exploration along these lines so that a strong inference may be drawn from any observations made. Thus, the plea for endosemiotics (Sebeok 1977) which I have strongly endorsed (Yates & Poston 1986) is not likely to move biologists, who are committed to experiment rather than to theory. The history of their subject has cautioned them against theorizing ahead of the availability of experimental data that could possibly check the theory.

9. Endosemiotics

Endosemiotics, as I employ the term, refers to chemical communications within or between multicellular living systems, and includes pharmacosemiotics. It is the province of semiotics overall to deal with messages – any messages whatsoever. The subject has been defined by Sebeok (1977: 1056) as follows:

> Since every message is composed of signs according to some ordered selection, semiotics has been variously identified as the doctrine or science, or the theory of signs. Correspondingly, the study designated semiotics comprises

> the set of general principles that underlie the structure of all signs, constituting a code, which was defined by Cherry as an agreed transformation, or set of unambiguous rules, whereby messages are converted from one representation to another ... Semiotics is concerned, successively, with the generation and encoding of messages, their propagation in any appropriate form of physical energy, their decoding and interpretation.

Messages require rules at both the transmission end (in this case, in the therapeutic system) and at the receiving end (the patient), and the rules must be matched appropriately for communication, control or command to occur. These rules are commonly syntactical and are not physical laws. They are local, arbitrary, and may be changed. The "meaning of a message" does not reside in a transmitted signal, which is purely a physical manifestation without semantic content. Meaning is found in the receipt of a message in the context of the receiver. The context of the receiver is established by: (1) the states of its memory; (2) the current dynamical state of the system; (3) its recent past dynamical states as they influence the current dynamical state; and (4) by the constraints it imposes on physical laws to create its local rules. Thus, the arrival of a message can either provoke or evoke responses; or it can merely change state transition probabilities – the dynamic contingencies – instead of the ongoing processes. We can never be certain that a cell did not receive a meaningful message just because we fail to see it do anything different after the message was transmitted. Unless we know the cellular "context", we cannot be sure about "interpretations" of chemical messages. About this difficulty I commented elsewhere (Yates 1981: 89):

> It is likely that we shall discover only the obvious messages, those that cause an immediate change in observable behavior. But we must never forget that meaningful messages change contingencies as well as processes, and the former, though perhaps unobservable, may be more important in the life of a cell ... To get at meanings, we shall have to decide how many different modes of behavior and how many internal states a receiving cell can have. My guess is that the number in each case will be relatively small (< 10), but different for different specialized cells ... We may find in endocrine signals the use of very functional commands ... Patterns of concentration in plasma may ultimately be interpreted as a broad command for a cell to divide. Or the message may be: "grow!" or "secrete!" We need to find out what aspect of concentration level is the essential part of the functional command. What we learn from such studies, if they are undertaken systematically, would have a potentially profound effect on the design of dosage forms and delivery systems.

10. Summary

Modern pharmacological research is intensely reductionistic, but the reductionistic program does not imply a constructionist program. Matching drugs to their receptors, either as agonists or antagonists, does not provide sufficient technical basis for predicting drug effects. Drug effects must always be found out by bioassay, including clinical trials. Presumably that situation will never change, but we might hope for better ways to determine efficacious and toxic effects of drug candidates, and the likelihood of occurrence in particular individuals. To do so would require better understanding the context of the system receiving the drug. That context is multidimensional and has a large parameter space, yet its operations are highly constrained. These constraints reduce the possibilities for drug action to a relatively small number of functional commands. The messages provided by drugs are conveyed by levels, rates of change and oscillatory phases (of concentrations). Biological messages are rarely conveyed by steady-state phenomena. Steadiness is death. Unfortunately, almost all current pharmacological dose-response data are presented as of the steady-state character. An expansion of pharmacological research from pharmacokinetics and pharmacodynamics to the conceptually richer pharmacosemiotics holds promise for providing clues that can optimize drug inputs, more efficiently to carry out the intentions of the prescribing physician.

References

Ariens, E. J.

1979 "Receptors: from fiction to fact", *Trends in Pharmacological Science* (TIPS) 1, 11–14.

Ayala, Francisco J.

1987 "Biological reductionism: the problems and some answers", in: F. Eugene Yates (ed.), 315–324.

Casti, John L. & A. Karlquist (eds.)

1985 *Complexity, language, and life: the mathematical approaches.* Berlin: Springer-Verlag.

Clynes, Manfred

1961 "Unidirectional rate sensitivity: A biocybernetic law of reflex and humeral systems as physiologic channels of control and communication", *Annals of the New York Academy of Science* 92, 946–969.

1962 "The non-linear biological dynamics of unidirectional rate sensitivity illustrated by analog computer analysis, pupilary reflex to light and sound, and heart rate behavior", *Annals of the New York Academy of Science* 98, 806–845.

Darnell, James, Harvey Lodish, & David Baltimore
1986 "Molecular cell biology", in: *Cell-to-cell signaling: hormones and receptors*. Scientific American Books. New York: W. H. Freeman, 667–714

Ehrlich, Paul
1913 "Chemotherapeutics: scientific principles, methods and results", *Lancet* 2, 445.

Garfinkel, Alan
1987 "The slime mold dictyostelium as a model of self-organization in social systems", in: F. Eugene Yates (ed.), 181–212.

Gilman, Alfred G., Louis S. Goodman, Theodore W. Rall & Ferid Murad
1985 *The pharmacological basis of therapeutics*. (7th edition.) New York: Macmillan Publishing Company, 35–48

Goldberger, Robert F.(ed.)
1982 *Biological regulation and development*. Vol. 3A. New York: Plenum Press.

Goldstein, Avram, Lewis Aronow & Sumner M. Kalman
1974 "Molecular mechanisms of drug action", in *Principles of drug action: the basis of pharmacology*. (2nd edition). New York: John Wiley and Sons, 1–127

Halberg, Franz
1969 "Chronobiology", *Annual Review of Physiology* 31, 675–725.

Kleene, S.C.
1952 *Introduction to mathematics*. New York: von Nostrand.

Kochen, Manfred & Harold M. Hastings (eds.)
1988 *Advances in cognitive science: steps toward convergence*. AAAS Selected Symposia Series, 104. Boulder CO: Westview Press.

Langley, John Newport
1909 "On the contraction of muscle, chiefly in relation to the presence of 'receptive' substances", Part IV. "The effect of curare and some other substances on the nicotine response of the sartorius and gastrocnemius muscles of the frog", *Journal of Physiology* 39, 235.

Lerner, R.M., D.F. Hultsch & R.A. Dixon
1983 "Contextualism and the character of developmental psychology in the 1970s", *Annals of the New York Academy of Sciences* 412, 101–128.

Lewin, Kurt
1935 "The conflict between Aristotelian and Galilean modes of thought in

contemporary psychology", in: *A dynamic theory of personality: selected papers*. New York: McGraw-Hill, 1–42

Pattee, Howard H.

1977 "Dynamic and linguistic modes of complex systems", International *Journal of General Systems* 3, 259–266.

1978 "The complementarity principle in biological and social structures", *Journal of Social and Biological Structures* 1, 191–200.

1982 "Cell psychology: an evolutionary approach to the symbol-matter problem. *Cognition and Brain Theory* 5, 325–341.

1985 "Universal principles of measurement and language functions in evolving systems", in: John L. Casti & A. Karlquist (eds.), 268–281.

1987 "Instabilities and information in biological self-organization", in: F. Eugene Yates (ed.), 325–338.

Pepper, Stephen C.

1942 *World hypotheses*. Berkeley CA: University of California Press.

Rosen, Robert

1986 "On the scope of syntactics in mathematics and science: the machine metaphor"; "Biology and physics: an essay in natural philosophy"; "Causal structures in brains and machines"; "On complex systems." [Four preprints available from the author at the Department of Physiology and Biophysics, Dalhousie University, Nova Scotia, Canada.]

Sebeok, Thomas A.

1977 "Zoosemiotic components of human communication", in: Thomas A. Sebeok (ed.), 1055–1077.

1987 "Participant in 'Semiotics and education: a dialogue'", Seminar series published by the Claremont Graduate School, Claremont, California, 13–14.

Sebeok, Thomas A. (ed.)

1977 *How animals communicate. Bloomington* in: Indiana University Press.

Struyker-Boudier, H.A.J. (ed.)

1986 *Principles and applications of rate-controlled drug administration and action*. Boca Raton FL: CRC Press.

Tomkins, Gordon N.

1975 "The metabolic code", *Science* 189, 760.

Weil, Andrew

1972 *The natural mind: a new way of looking at drugs and the higher consciousness*. Boston MA: Houghton-Mifflin Co.

Yates, F. Eugene

1979 "Integrative pharmacology – beyond structure-activity relationships into

pharmacolinguistics", *American Journal of Physiology: Regulatory, Integrative and Comparative Physiology* 6, 251–253.
1981 "Analysis of endocrine signals: the engineering and physics of biochemical communication systems", *Biology of Reproduction* 24, 73–94.
1982 "Systems analysis of hormone action: principles and strategies", in: Robert F. Goldberger (ed.), 25–97.
1985 "Semiotics as bridge between information (biology) and dynamics (physics)", *Recherches Sémiotiques/Semiotic Inquiry* 5, 347–360.
1987 "Quantumstuff and biostuff: a view of patterns of convergence in contemporary science", epilogue to F. Eugene Yates (ed.), 617–644.
1988 "Evolutionary computing by dynamics in living organisms", in: Manfred Kochen & Harold M. Hastings (eds.), 26–49.

Yates, F. Eugene (ed.)
1987 *Self-organizing systems: the emergence of order*. New York: Plenum Press.

Yates, F. Eugene & Peter N. Kugler
1984 "Signs, singularities and significance: a physical model for semiotics", *Semiotica* 52, 49–77.

Yates, F. Eugene & Timothy Poston
1986 "Rate-controlled delivery of endocrine agents: some paradoxical consequences of controlling the inputs", in: H.A.J. Struyker-Boudier (ed.), 247–272.

Elements of semiotic theory relevant to psychoanalysis

Bonnie E. Litowitz

Introduction

Semiotics has its etymological roots in Ancient Greece (το σημα 'sign'; σημαινω 'to give a sign') where the presentation of signs (from the Latin, *signum*) and their interpretation were important to medicine, religion and warfare. Because man does not directly signal his intention of love or aggression as do other animals, soldiers on watch demand a sign to distinguish friend from foe. Man's Gods have always communicated with him indirectly through the use of signs and several religions proscribe specific types of signs – e.g., one can talk about God but not make graven images or use His real name; one can create images in Islamic art but not literal representations of any living thing. Critical to medical diagnosis has always been the reading of signs that indicate sickness or health.

The fact that man does not indicate this intentions, needs, states of illness or well-being directly, but rather through signs, has led theorists to the study of the nature of signs, their uses and principles of interpretation. Since early times these theorists have come from diverse fields in which signs figure prominently, e.g., philosophy, linguistics, psychology, medicine, literary studies, anthropology. The history of contributions to semiotics consists of specific philosophers, linguists, etc. who have chosen to address these issues. Only very recently has a discipline of semiotics *per se*, complete with semioticians arisen to create a general theory or metatheory of signs. Some semioticians distinguish this general metatheory of semiotics relevant to any discussion of signs in whatever field from specific theories such as medical semiotics, zoological semiotics or even psychoanalytic semiotics (Pelc 1981; Bruss 1980).

In what follows I will first address general principles of semiotics, presenting what we know about that part of signs in general that is relevant to psychoanalysis in particular. Then I will apply this background to a reinterpretation of three critical concepts – symptoms, dreams and discourse. Hopefully, it will be clear that what one gains from semiotics is not a new theory of psychoanalysis but rather a new perspective on the data that one gathers as a psychoanalyst and on the theories used to explain them.

1. Semiotics

The basic premise of a semiotic perspective is, as illustrated in the opening examples, that man can only know his world indirectly. Man's knowledge is not immediate, a direct copy or presentation of reality. Rather, his knowledge is mediated or re-presented. Thus, between reality and knowledge a gap or space occurs; and out of that gap, interpretation arises. In other words, if reality and our knowledge of it were one and the same, we would never need to ask: what does it mean (where "it" refers to picture, word or any kind of sign)? (See figure 1.)

knowledge = mediated, indirect, re-presentation of reality

knowledge 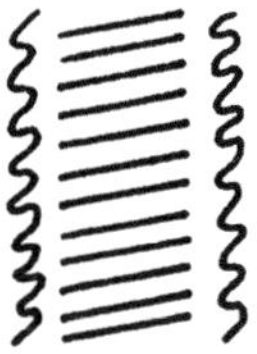 reality

Figure 1: The relationship between knowledge and reality

Although several philosophers and linguistics had addressed the nature of signs in language before de Saussure (Mueller-Vollmer 1986), he made a definition of verbal signs fundamental to the newly developing science of linguistics (1959). He stated that linguistics is the study of verbal signs and thereby a subcategory of semiology, the study of signs in general.

In banning all other signs from his inquiry, de Saussure's privileging of the linguistic system had several consequences.[1] The most important for us is the cutting off of language from other sign systems, leaving Saussurean analysis of the verbal sign insufficient to explain sign phenomena that are non-linguistic, but clearly semiotic. The two major areas where this deficit emerges most profoundly are in studies of the development of representational abilities in infants and children, itself an aspect of the development of knowledge (or intelligence); and in psychological investigations such as psychoanalysis. Obviously, children are born *infantis* but not without nonverbal signaling behaviors. As we shall see, psychoanalysis addresses a wide range of semiosis. Both areas share a need to address the relationship of language to prelingual, non-lingual, and paralingual representations, as these change over time. Thus, de Saussure's separation of synchronic/structural analysis from diachronic history renders Saussurean semiotics additionally problematic.[2]

Every psychological theory, each in its own way, has to address issues of the representation of knowledge, as can be seen in: Piaget's semiotic function (1951);

Vygotsky's semiotic mediation (1978; Wertsch 1983); distributed memories of information processing models (Neisser 1967); and most recently, cognitive science. Psychoanalysis is distinguished from other psychological theories at least in three respects for which semiotics is pertinent: the distinction between instinct (or need) and wish (or desire); the positing of unconscious knowledge; and a genetic perspective that links early experiences to later behavior. We will return to these points below.

But first, what is a sign – the basic unit of semiosis (representation)? A sign is most simply something that stands for or re-presents something else in some way to someone. De Saussure has given us a set of labels for the first two parts of that basic definition: something and something else. That which represents is the *signifier* and what is represented is the *signified*. The purpose of these terms is to make it easier to talk about two necessary aspects of any sign. De Saussure used a simple linguistic example to illustrate: the word *tree* consists of an acoustic image *[tri]* – a sequence of three phonemes, its signifier – representing the concept of 'tree' as its signified, for which de Saussure provided a line drawing of an idealized tree. How this signifier came to be connected to this signified for a specific individual, or whether the signified is in fact an idealized image, a real tree or another word, and whether we share prototypical images as we do words, etc. – these are questions de Saussure does not address. He only goes on to say that, as for language, the relationship between signifier and signified is totally arbitrary (i.e., artificial and not naturally occurring) and, therefore, conventional and social. Obviously, the concept of tree is represented by *arbre* in French, *Baum* in German, and so forth. (See figure 2.)

sign = something that represents something else in some way to someone

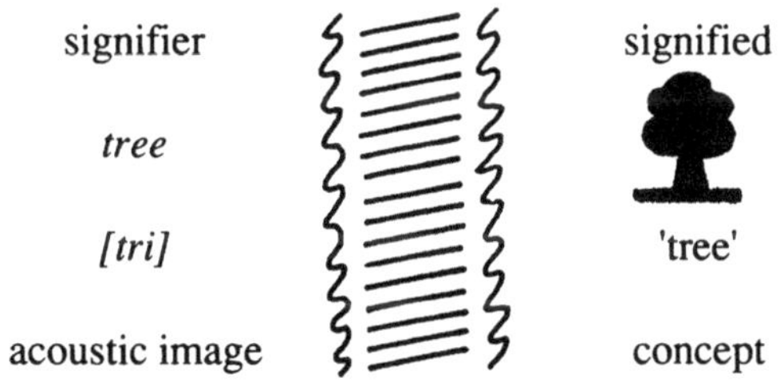

Figure 2: One definition of a sign: de Saussure

Now, the problems that arise from Saussurean semiology at this point are twofold. While there is a gap between signifier and signified, there is no need for interpretation since connections are conventionally set and socially shared. On this view, to know a language is in part to know its signifier-signified equivalences. Indeed, this sense of definition as logical equivalence remains a feature of formal semantics rendering it of little value to a psychoanalytic psychology. This misconception is due to the second problem, an exclusion of the two qualifying phrases in our basic sign definition: (something that stands for or represents something else) in some way; to some one. To address these aspects we must turn to Peirce (1931–1958; 1955).

Unlike de Saussure whose goal was to delimit the boundaries of a legitimate science of language, Charles Sanders Peirce, an American pragmatist-philosopher, elaborated arguably the most influential theory of semiotics as part of a larger programme for the philosophy of science, specifically in regard to epistemology or the study of knowledge. Whereas de Saussure's aim was to exclude all but the verbal sign, Peirce's goal was to explain the properties and principles of all signs by means of a calculus of relations. Towards that end, he set up a series of multiple triads[3] that, when fully elaborated, would create a net of cross-classifications into which any sign would fall. A given sign, then, could be fully defined by its position of interlocking relationships.[4] (See figure 3.)

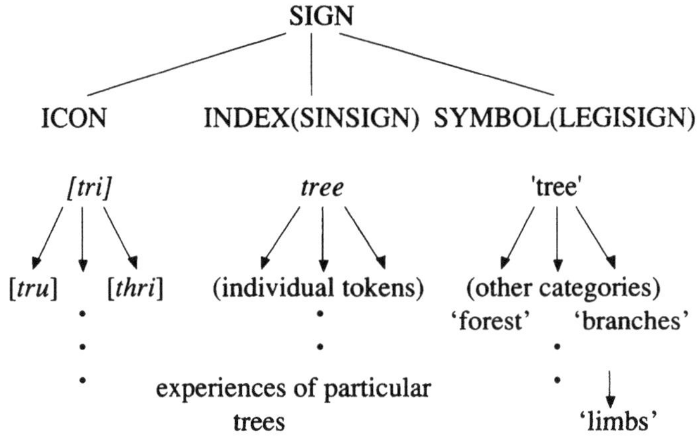

Figure 3: Another definition of a sign: Peirce

Peirce's contribution is his focus on the two qualifying phrases of our (actually, his) definition. He emphasizes that signs are not static equivalences but are first and foremost the result of an act of interpretation. The most common mistake of novice semioticians is to view the relationship of signifier to signified as fixed, objective and external; that is, existing in the real world by virtue of the type of sign involved, when in fact it is always imposed upon reality by an act of interpretation.

The source of this error can be clearly seen in de Saussure who emphasizes words *as* signs. In contrast, Peirce would claim that words can be – even, are most often – interpreted as symbols, by which he means as arbitrary, conventional and socially determined. Still, at the same time, other kinds of interpretations are potentially available for words. Words have an iconic form – a sound and shape – and they index or point to other signs.

To see how cross-classifications can illuminate the subtleties of signs, take de Saussure's example of *tree*. *Tree* is a symbol (i.e., a Saussurean sign) in that its meaning is socially fixed; it is a sign by law or a *legisign*. As such, a symbol always represents a class, a category or a type, not a particular instance or token of that class. Most people are unaware that when they say *tree* they refer to a class or category which needs to be made specific by use of an additional sign, an index (*sinsign*): *the tree*, *a tree*, *that tree*. We tend to overlook or look through these indexical signs that tie a symbol to its specific circumstances. Yet, our experience with trees is always through a particular one, a token of that type. Even every time we say [*tri*] is a unique instantiation of a class of acoustic images, or what Peirce calls a *sinsign* for single sign. Thus a sign that is socially shared can also represent an individual, single (particular) experience with that sign – a fact that is very important to understanding how symbols are used in dreams. Dreams use word-symbols in their iconic and indexical manifestations, e.g., the homonymic/homophonic associations and words actually spoken in dreams.[5]

We understand the meaning of a sign as a choice among the iconic, indexical and symbolic aspects of the sign, as well as through its relationships to other signs. In our example, we chose *tree* but not *true* or *three* which sounds similar; having chosen *tree* we are connected to *forest* as 'a collection of trees' or to *branches* and *limbs* (or *leaves* and *bark*) as 'parts of trees', and so forth. In other words, we find that the meaning of a sign is always another sign – in an endless signifying chain.

In discourse, in dreams, in schizophrenia, in poetry, in word magic or in children's talk, different aspects of this representational richness is available or brought into focus. We interpret one and the same sign differently in each context. Some of us even interpret one and the same sign differently in the same context, e.g., a paranoid, an hysteric, a neurotic. The interpretation we make is the new knowledge that emerges from retracing all the interconnections and aspects mentioned above and the awareness that in choosing one aspect, others were denied. It is not an equivalence but rather the play of the differences among all the semiotic potentialities. This is why we say that the presence of a sign is also an absence. First, it stands for something not present; and second, its presence implies all the others not chosen (absent). As Peirce claims: a sign is something by knowing which we know something more (1931–58, 8: 332). We know all that it is not.

It may seem that Peirce's symbols are just another way to address de Saussure's signs, albeit with slightly more elaboration. To see that this is not so let me take one more example: *I*. *I*, like *tree*, is a word and therefore a *legisign*, but it functions as an indexical sign because, unlike *tree*, *I* does not represent a class. Rather, it serves only to point out whosoever is speaking. As soon as the speaker changes, the referent for *I* shifts. As mentioned earlier, there are many indexical words whose function is to tie language to particular contexts or to indicate something about language itself. These words seem to have considerable psychological sig-ni-ficance as evidenced by: the difficulties psychotic children have in mastering *I* and *you*; the time it takes normal children to acquire *I* in spite of its frequent use (Litowitz & Litowitz 1983); the shift from I to *you/he/they* in stress or paranoia.

It has become increasingly commonplace to hear about this "I" as the speaking subject, as authors focus on the conflict between shifting indicator (index) and our need for a more permanent sense of self. Again, development is important here. What sense of self do children have before "I" (at the end of the second/beginning of the third year)? Lacan's answer, based on a mirror-stage, is one based on images – the imaginary – superimposed later by the symbolic "I" (1977).

One last set of terms, more familiar than some mentioned, is useful to any discussion of semiotics. When speaking of the meanings of signs we are addressing *semantics*, the relation of signs to what they represent. Signs also combine in an ordered sequence which is called *syntax* and whose rules comprise a grammar. A word does not occur alone in a sentence, embodying a proposition. While language is always linear, visual images can be simultaneously presented, as in dreams. This is why dreams have a different syntax or grammar. Lastly, *pragmatics* is the relation of signs to their users or interpreters (Morris 1938). (See figure 4.)

2. Psychoanalysis

Let us now turn to psychoanalysis, examining it as a semiotic enterprise. If we assume that psychoanalysis seeks to understand individual meanings, the relevance of semiotics to psychoanalysis should be clear. As we have seen, those meanings are represented by varied sign relationships, many of which were in turn acquired during periods of developing abilities to represent knowledge. Psychoanalysis takes as axiomatic that knowledge is mediated, that one's perception of reality is filtered according to a particular state of psychic need and at a particular developmental phase. Every case study and clinical example in Freud's work is a testament to the primacy of the interpretation of signs in psychoanalysis: symptom as sign; dream as sign; and language as sign. Unfortunately, Freud lacked a unifying theory of semiosis and used instead the more limiting metaphor of language:

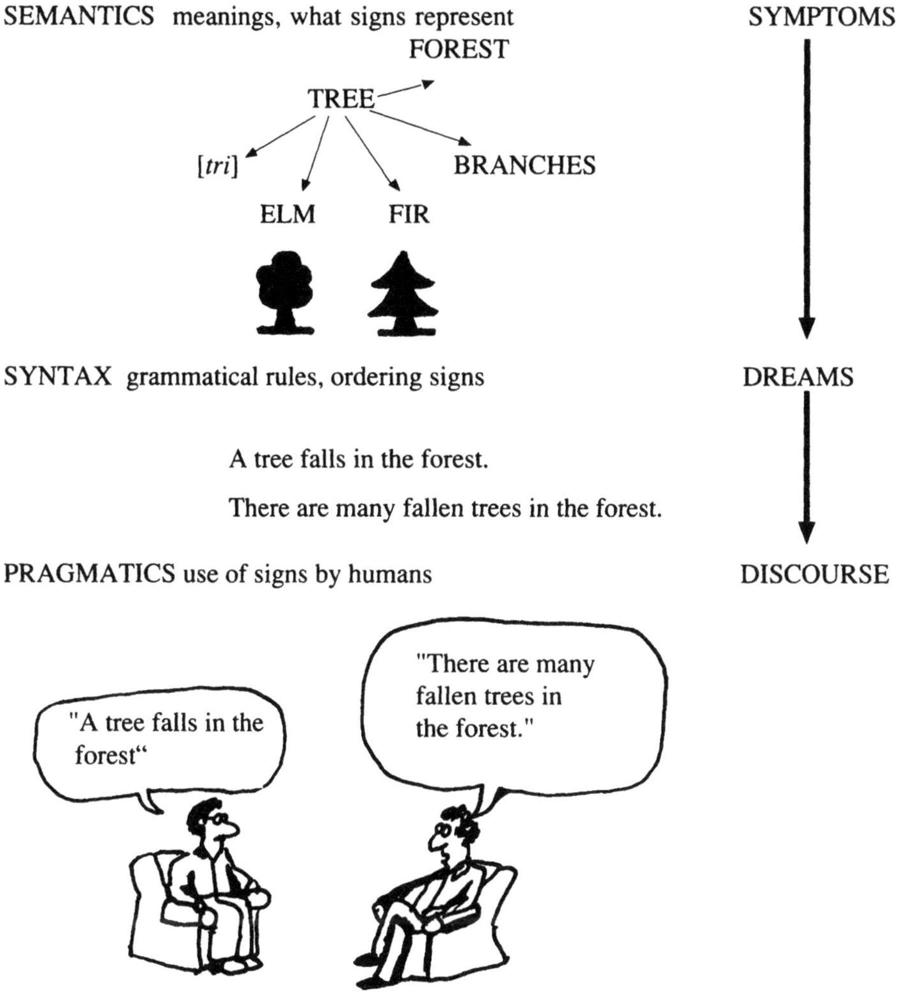

Figure 4: Three branches of semiotics

the unconscious speaks more than one dialect. According to the differing psychological conditions governing and distinguishing the various forms of neurosis, we find regular modifications in the way in which unconscious mental impulses are expressed. While the gesture-language of hysteria agrees on the whole with the picture-language of dreams and visions, etc., the thought-language of obsessional neurosis and of the paraphrenias (dementia praecox and paranoia) exhibits special idiomatic peculiarities which,

> in a number of instances, we have been able to understand and interrelate. For instance,what an hysteric expresses by vomiting an obsessional will express by painstaking protective measures against infection, while a paraphrenic will be led to complaints or suspicions that he is being poisoned. These are all of them *different* representations of the patient's wish to become pregnant which have been repressed into the unconscious, or of his defensive reaction against that wish (1913: 178). [Emphasis added]

We now understand that "different representations" refers to different kinds of signs (rather than dialectal variants of one language), but let us address what is represented: the wish. Energy manifests itself in human psychology in the form of instincts or instinctual impulses (instincts in action) that define our needs and as such are shared with other animals (e.g., needs for reproduction, satisfaction, self-preservation). In humans, however, these needs are always attached or bound to a representation (*Vorstellungsrepräsentanz*) – a thing, an idea, a memory – which Freud calls the "wish" or "desire". Thus emerges in Freudian theory, in its very foundations, the same semiotic gap of mediation and representation that necessitates interpretation. Just as knowledge is always separated from reality and sign from what it represents (signifier from signified), desire or wish is always separated from instinctual need. And further, just as we perceive the sign as the thing for which it stands, we experience our desires as real needs. Lacan (1977) is the first, to my knowledge, to refocus our attention on this gap and to create one more turn on it in addressing the articulation of desire in language as yet an additional gap of "demand". That is, when expressed as "I want", a speaking subject "I" uses language composed of signifiers distanced from their signifieds to represent a wish that is in turn a mediated need. Further, the speaking subject thinks he is real (when in fact he is alienated: but that's another story) and that his need is real, instinctual. To truly understand who he is and what he wants requires the unraveling of multiple acts of interpretation, and those unravelings are themselves acts of interpretation. (See figure 5.)

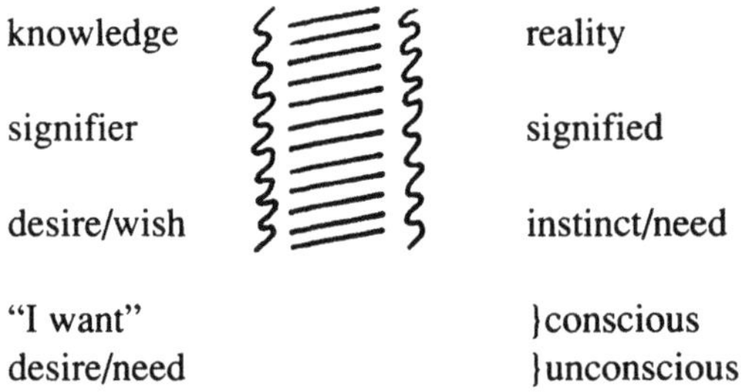

Figure 5: Figures 1 and 2 revisited

2.1 *Symptoms*

Before there was theory, however, there were patients and symptoms: aphasics who could not speak; hysterics who could not walk or raise a hand or see; neurasthenics with shifting bodily sensations, night terrors, and phobias; obsessives with repetitious words and images. Freud had to look at these phenomena, "till [as he says of Charcot] his repeated and unbiased efforts allowed him to reach a correct view of its meaning" (1885: 10). The reading of symptoms as signs is the most basic act of interpretation in medicine or any healing art. The symptom is always at least an indexical sign whose function is to direct attention to a past cause or a future consequence (Baer 1982). In purely physical disease processes, the relationship between signifier and signified is close: abdominal pain indicates peritonitis; peritonitis indicates an infection of the peritoneum; and that infection indicates a ruptured appendix; and so forth. In psychogenic disease processes such as in neurosis, however, abdominal pain may represent something else and not necessarily primarily as an index. For example: it could represent an hysterical identification with someone who suffers from abdominal disorders, like an icon which is similar to what it represents because it shares some quality; it could represent labor and the wish to be pregnant. In psychological cases, Freud notes, "a symptom is a sign of, and a substitute for, an instinctual satisfaction which has remained in abeyance; it is a consequence of the process of repression" (1926: 91).

The sign always makes present again (re-presents) something (in the examples just given, a person or a wish) that is absent but does so only indirectly. Unlike natural signs, the relationship between the signs as a natural indication of the fact of labor and the use of these to symbolize a counterfactual wish – that is, the wish to be pregnant when one is not – cannot be discovered through iconic resemblance, natural indication or consensual agreement. This particular symptom is created through an act of interpretation by the neurotic (unconsciously, of course) and it can only be understood – what does the stomach pain mean to this patient – by patient and therapist. (I will return to joint-interpretation below in discussing discourse.)

Freud's earliest writings attempt to differentiate psychological illnesses and to distinguish one such illness from another (e.g., hysteria from anxiety, neurosis from obsession) by virtue of how each illness' symptoms are formed. These differences turn out to be largely representational. For example, in anxiety neurosis the anxiety may be expresses directly without ideational content (i.e., an anxiety attack) or may be "accompanied by the interpretation that is nearest to hand" (1926: 91). The "patient picks out in particular now one, now another, factor" (1895b: 94). These, then, are the presenting symptoms of the anxiety neurosis which may be similar to those in hysterical and in obsessional neuroses. That is, both anxiety and obsessional neurotics may present phobias, but the choice in the former case does not include substitution of the phobia for a repressed idea and, therefore, is "not amenable to psycho-therapy" because it is "not reducible by psycho-logical analysis" (1895b: 97). In other words, phobia in the anxiety neurotic cannot be traced back through substitutions of signifiers and signifieds; there was no act of interpretation in its choice.[6]

Similarly, in distinguishing hysterical from organic paralysis, Freud notes that organic paralysis is determined solely by neuroanatomy whereas hysterical paralysis is determined by the patient's knowledge of anatomy:

> in its paralyses and other manifestations hysteria behaves as though anatomy did not exist or *as though it had no knowledge of it* ... it has no knowledge of the optic chiasma, and consequently it does not produce hemianopsia. *It takes the organs in the ordinary, popular sense of the names they bear*: The leg is the leg as far up as its insertion into the hip, the arm is the upper limb as it is visible under the clothing. There is no reason for adding paralysis of the face to paralysis of the arm. An hysteric who cannot talk has no motive for forgetting his understanding of speech (1893: 169). [Emphasis added]

In these descriptions we see patients' active (motivated) creation of symptoms based on linguistic knowledge, in this case names of body parts. We share with the patients part of that knowledge: a leg is a limb or bodily extremity whose function is for standing upright, locomotion. The use of a leg as symptom, however, forces us to seek additional meaning. In asking, "why a leg?", we are asking both: (1) what does leg stand for – what absent idea, thing, wish is allowed to be present through this symptom (i.e., what is it a sign of?); and (2) why is this sign written on the body and not represented in verbal parapraxis, the visual imagery of dreams, an obsessionally repeated thought? Why this kind of a sign and not another?

Freud offers many examples of signs created out of linguistic knowledge, the meanings of which are inaccessible (because of repression) to the sign-creator who can rediscover their meaning with the help of a sign-reader. The shared linguistic knowledge acts as an entry point to this joint project. The oft-analyzed *Herr-signore – Botticelli – Signorelli* example (1898: 287–97; see Baer 1974; Schimek 1974; Wilden 1972) is producible and understandable, as Eco points out, "only by someone who knows both German and Italian" (1984: 24). But a knowledge of German and Italian alone cannot let you interpret this *Fehlleistung*. The shift in the auditory surface of words is created along a line of displacement; and "the line of displacement was laid down by the names that were contained in the repressed topic" (Freud 1898: 293), substituted names of provinces and painters. And only the creator of this compromise formation knows these connections. Other examples from *Introductory lectures on psycho-analysis* (Freud 1916–1917), *Studies on hysteria* (Breuer & Freud 1893–1895), *The interpretation of dreams* (Freud 1900), *The psychopathology of everyday life* (Freud 1901b), and elsewhere are too numerous to mention.

The overriding point is that Freud's many examples depend upon a theory of knowledge as mediated by different signs out of which a new sign is created in compromise formations such as dreams, parapraxes, and symptoms. These new signs are always overdetermined in that: (1) they include both unconscious and conscious information; and (2) they are never the result of a simple equivalence or a single natural connection. Rather, these signs result from several elements intertwined and interconnected, arising out of the whole fabric from which they are woven. Created by an act of interpretation, their meanings can only be unraveled in another act of interpretation within the psychoanalytic discourse.

In summary, psychological symptoms are similar to physical symptoms in that they index or point to a disease process. They differ from physical symptoms in that they are always representational and mediational. In the gap that occurs between created sign and its meaning there is a great deal of room for variation according to individual expression of desires, which unlike the expression of physical illness, is always counterfactual and intentional. An understanding of the differences in sign formations leads to an appreciation of the differences among psychological illnesses and even to the transformations possible within any one illness (e.g., within obsessional neurosis, 1896: 169–71).

An appreciation of the multiplicity of sign phenomena and their transformations has set Freudian psychology apart from other psychologies from its beginnings, and has added to our understanding of sign relationships. *The Project for a scientific psychology* (1895a: 281) had already described simple connections between word-representations and thing-representations: signifier-signified. But later, in an appendix to "The unconscious" (1915: 209) Freud elaborated a semiotic complex around the word-representation (*Wortvorstellung*) that includes various 'images' (*Bild*): visual; motoric; acoustic. These images connect to various object-associations: visual; tactile; acoustic. This basic notion of representational-associational networks is augmented by descriptions of thematic-associational connections, described, for example, in *The studies on hysteria* (Breuer & Freud 1893–1895): relationships of similar time and space or of shared topic or property; connections of a chronological sequence; a dynamic zig-zag path of a peculiar kind of logic (Litowitz 1978). In this way, we see that Freud had a more sophisticated notion of representation than the limited linguistic one of signifier (word) and signified (thing). (See figure 6.)

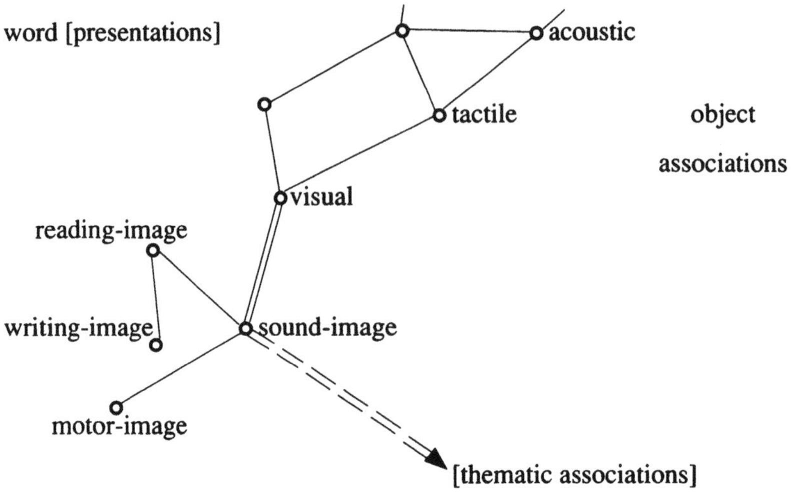

Figure 6: From Freud's Appendix C to "The unconscious" (S.E. XIV: 214) Sigmund Freud Copyrights, the Institute of Psycho-Analysis and The Hogarth Press.

Throughout his writing, Freud gave copious examples of the shifts among these elements of representation and the peculiar logic that they obey. In spite of changes in metapsychology, Freud's writing remains fresh and compelling in large part because of his careful and detailed presentation of these clinical examples: what the patient actually said; the dream images and their verbal associations as reported by the patient.

2.2 *Dreams*

Although not the earliest description of the semantics and syntax of sign phenomena in Freud's work, *The interpretation of dreams* (1900) is certainly the richest. Freud used the decipherment of the dream as illustrative of unconscious semiotic elaboration and primary process logic. Not the only road to this knowledge, it is however the "royal" one. Freud notes that it is "only the first to be discovered of a whole series of psychical processes, responsible for the generation of hysterical symptoms, of phobias, obsessions, and delusions (as well as) a whole number of the phenomena of the everyday life of healthy people – such as forgetting, slips of the tongue, bungled actions and (other) errors ... " (1901a: 671). Mechanisms of the dreamwork, "condensation and, above all, displacement are invariable characteristics of these and other processes as well ... Modification into pictorial form, on the other hand, remains a peculiarity of the dream-work" (1901a: 671).

We all know how the dreamwork alters latent dream thoughts into visual pictorial images, "according to their symbolic relation" (1900: 277), i.e., as indirectly representing something else. Sometimes latent dream thoughts go through a prior translation into an intermediate, more readily pictured verbal form (1901a: 650). That intermediate form is already itself a construction by the dreamwork, usually a whole verbal phrase as complex sign. Even as it works with visual images, the dreamwork makes use of words since they are the nodal points of numerous ideas (1900: 340) and act as "switch-words" (1905: 65 fn, 82) connecting many lines of thought necessary to interpretation (see also 1900: 282–3).[7] The dream-work exploits verbal ambiguity, assonance and alliteration, etc.; that is, the auditory images of words or their iconic aspects: "the verbal malformations in dreams greatly resemble those which are familiar in paranoia but which are also present in hysteria and obsessions. The linguistic tricks performed by children who sometimes actually treat words as though they were objects and moreover invent new languages and artificial syntactic forms, are the common source of these things in dreams and psychoneuroses alike" (1900: 303).

Besides recalling our early childhood relations to verbal material, dreams also have access to material unchanged from childhood (1900: 589), both "impressive experiences ... perceived as a rule as situations having a visual subject-matter" (1901a: 659) and words whose childhood meanings differ from those of adults; for example, "a child's idea of being 'dead' has nothing much in common with ours apart from the word"(1900: 254). I will return shortly to these developmental questions.

2.3 Symbols

In addition to current and past experiences, images and words, the dreamwork has a stock of ready-to-hand symbols. Ironically, although Freud's discussion of symbols would seem to be the most directly semiotic material in his writing, it turns out to be the least interesting. Freud vacillated on the concept of symbols as fixed equivalences: x always represents y. His concept of symbol, fully elaborated by Jones, led him into murky Lamarckian waters of an inherited collective unconscious and to fuzzy speculations on an original *Ursprache* from which our Tower of Babel linguistic diversity descended (Litowitz & Litowitz 1977). This evolutionary journey must be repeated by each new unconscious; that is, not only does ontogeny recapitulate phylogeny but this history is still hanging around as *Ursprache*, providing the real and true meaning to our signs. Why exactly the older original equivalences are necessarily repressed would not clear unless they are part of our genetic endowment, as a part of our unconscious that is pregiven and not due to repression, i.e., the collective unconscious of our species.

On some level, Freud recognized the irony of turning away from ancient dreambook interpretations only to arrive at a new dreambook. Positing a small set of fixed signifier-signified equivalences (birth, death, genitals, etc.) renders the interpretation process at the very least boring, and at the very worst, a joke. If the end of every interpretive journey is to arrive back at the beginning (as Eliot says) and to know it for the first time, it does not necessarily follow that that beginning is the same for all travelers. It may be home or infantile wishes yet meaning lies not in reductive equivalences but arises from the many acts of interpretation that constitute the journey itself.

Freud's vacillation can be seen in his warning against expecting "that if we had a still profounder knowledge of dream-symbolism ... we could do without asking the dreamer for his associations to the dream and go back entirely to the technique of dream-interpretation of antiquity. Quite apart from individual symbols and oscillations in the use of universal ones, one can never tell whether any particular element in the content of a dream is to be interpreted symbolically (1901a: 684) ... or whether its interpretation is to depend on its wording ... whether it is to be taken in a positive or negative sense (as an antithetic relation) ... whether it is to be interpreted historically (as a recollection)" (1900: 341). He even allowed, on occasion, that symbols might be restricted to "a single linguistic or cultural group" (1901a: 684) or that "dreams are so closely related to linguistic expression that ... every tongue has its own dream-language" (1900: 99fn).

A strong position on the Freudian symbol contains two fallacies. First, the premise that one needs to use a symbol only to represent that which cannot be represented directly due to repression is clearly untenable. All knowledge is mediated and therefore capable of being symbolized; repressed knowledge undergoes further mediation – changes in representation due to compromise formations as Freud describes. Second, as many have pointed out, while biology obeys the principles of Darwinian evolution, culture is indeed Lamarckian, though not as Freud or Jung supposed. The meanings of symbols and other legisigns are social and collective; meanings acquired in one generation may indeed be passed on to the next. But as Freud noted above, these are only the raw material that can be used by an individual in many different ways.

2.4 Syntax

The syntax of unconscious representation is clearly elaborated by Freud. All the logical relations that exist between propositions and predicates (in the propositional and predicate calculi) are inoperative in the primary process with the exception of conjunction. It is analysis' role to reinstate the loss of these logical relations: disjunction, negation, material and strict (biconditional) implication (1900: 312 & 1901a: 660). The dream can reverse cause and effect, provide multiple and conflicting causes, or replace cause altogether with temporal/spatial juxtaposition or sequences. Negation does not exist, and and replaces or. Every language has indexical signs whose function is not to represent concepts, but rather, to connect and interrelate such representations (as we saw with *I* versus *tree*). It was to Freud's credit that he recognized that the dreamwork replaces these special verbal signs with unique forms, many of which are particular to the visual mode: foreground and background (1901a: 660) for focus and presupposition; tense and aspect by presence and simultaneity (1901a: 647); types are reduced to tokens; similars and partitives become synonyms; antonyms become synonyms (the dream prefers the "just-as" relation); grammatical relations such as agentive can become objective, and active voice can become passive (Litowitz 1977). (See figure 7.)

dream syntax (wishes):	language syntax (propositions):	
and	conjunction	*and*
and	disjunction	*or*
and	negation	*not*
and	implication	*if-then*
		if & only if-then
foreground & background	focus & presupposition	
	topic & comment	
presence & simultaneity	tense & aspect	
tokens & instances	types & categories	
synonyms	similars	
synonyms	partitives	
synonyms	antonyms	
altered grammatical relations	fixed relations	

Figure 7: The comparative syntactics of wishes and propositions

We see in the description of logic that underlies dreams and other psychic productions transformations between the syntax of wishes and the syntax of propositions. For example, Little Hans' neurosis did not consist in merely substituting a horse for his father, although Freud claims: "what made it a neurosis was one thing alone: the replacement of his father by a horse. It is this displacement, then, which has a claim to be called a symptom" (1926: 103). The displacement is just the beginning, however, and would result only in Hans' wanting to kill horses. Instead,

Hans was afraid that horses would bite him. Thus, rather than express himself as the agent of aggression, he became its object: I want to kill my father –> my father wants to harm me –> horses want to bite me. Such syntactic transformations of desire were illustrated most clearly in the variety of permutations on the paranoiac, "I (a man) love him (a man)": he loves me; I hate him; he hates me; etc. (1911: 63–5).[8] One of Lacan's contributions to this syntax is his exploration of embedded desire: my desire is the desire of the other/my desire is the other's desire/my desire is that I am the desire of the other (1977). In other words, rather than just surface syntactic permutations, such embeddings point to deeper levels of the transformations of desire. (See figures 8 & 9.)

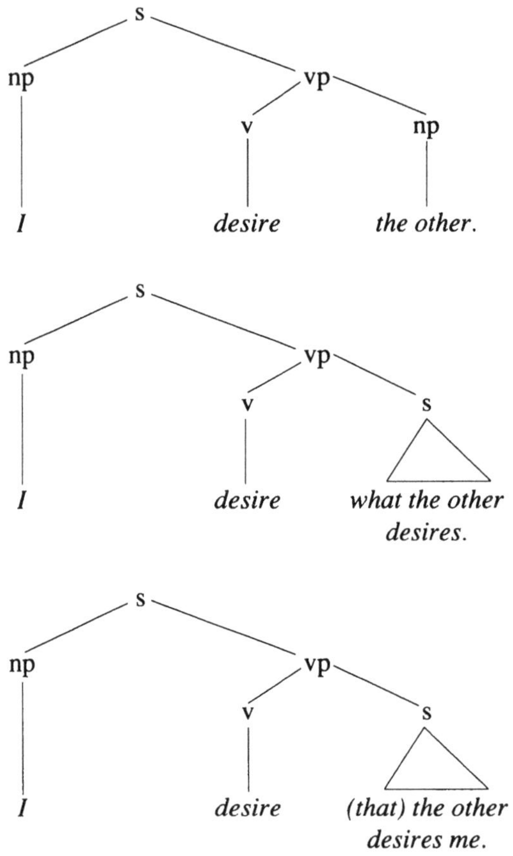

Figure 8: The embeddings of desire: propositions

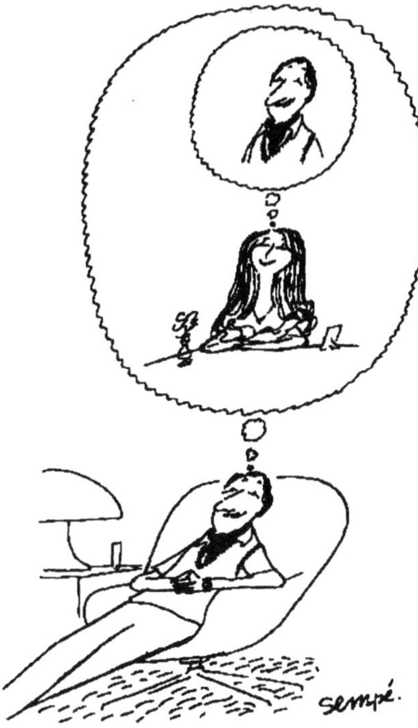

Figure 9: The embeddings of desire: wishes
Drawing by Sempé © 1985 The New Yorker Magazine, Inc.

By way of turning to development, I want now to call attention to a distinction that Freud makes between dreams and schizophrenia; and he does so on the basis of representation. In dreams there is a topographical regression to perception while in schizophrenia there is not (1917: 229). We may say that in dreams words are represented by the things they stand for, as written in a rebus from which we must reconstruct a text. (The translation analogy is often used.) In schizophrenia, words become things in and of themselves; they become only their own qualities because they lose their capacity as symbols. Freud says they are "cut off"; and Lacan claims they are "foreclosed". The effects of this cut are radical for psychoanalytic method. It becomes questionable whether such cases of psychosis are reducible by psychological analysis or amenable to psychotherapy. Recalling Freud's description of anxiety neurosis (1895b: 97), mentioned earlier, we may ask: are there illnesses which because of the nature of their representations are not analyzable?

In noting the topographical *regression* to perception in dreams, Freud is suggesting that some forms of representation, specifically visual images, are prior to other forms. The editors of the Standard Edition comment on three ways Freud used regression: (1) topographically, based on that early model in which psychical processes advanced from perception to motor discharge; (2) temporally, a return to earlier libidinal objects or earlier ways of functioning; and (3) formally, "where primitive methods of expression and representation take the place of the usual ones (1895a: 344–6). In 1914, however, Freud commented on these uses: "All these three kinds of regression are, however, one at bottom and occur together as a rule; for what is older in time is more primitive in form and in psychical topography lies nearer to the perceptual end" (1900: 548). In other words, "dreaming is on the whole an example of regression to the dreamer's earliest condition, a revival of his childhood, of the instinctual impulses which dominated it and of the methods of expression which were then available to him" (1900: 548).[9]

3. Development

Freud here raises a question pertinent to semiotics that is empirically testable: Is there a developmental sequence of representational capacities such that one form of sign can be said to be more primitive? The answer, I think, is yes, but not necessarily as Freud envisioned it. I will give three possible responses.

Bruner (1973) suggests that there are three basic ways of representing the world as knowledge: enactive, iconic and symbolic. These are operative for the infant and young child in that order and are additive, with earlier ways remaining throughout life, and with the potential to transform information from one representational form into another. That is, what we learn visually we can talk about or what we learn verbally we can enact. Using this view, regression to actions would be more primitive than to images, as in dreams. Regression could activate memories that are still encoded enactively or iconically; or could cause a return to a way of representing that was prevalent at an earlier age.

Piaget (1951) elaborates a sequence of representational ability based on a merger of Saussurean and Peircean semiotics. The infant begins with signals and progresses to indices, images, symbols, and signs (in that order), thereby gaining greater and greater distance between signifiers and signifieds. Dreams make use of symbols which embody motivated, idiosyncratic signifier-signified relationships, and which remain available in dreams throughout life.[10] The ability to use arbitrary, conventional signs (i.e., completely distanced signifier-signified) begins around 2 years, is designated by Piaget as the semiotic (or symbolic) function, and takes some time to develop fully. For Piaget, this function is manifested in all kinds of representational or figurative intelligence: perception, memory, language, drawing and play. Such figurative intelligence develops as a reflection of operational knowledge (mathematico-logical structures).

Therefore, regression, on this view, would imply both a different point in representational capacity and a different organization of knowledge. Such knowledge would be precausal, favoring instead syncretism, juxtaposition and transduction. Freud gives a good example of this type of thinking in his description of the creation of hysterical symptoms (Breuer & Freud 1893–1895: 212, 175) or of his multiple and contradictory excuses in the Irma Dream (Freud 1900: 119).

Like other developmentalists, Vygotsky (1962; 1978) is concerned about the growth and changes in representational knowledge. Even more than for Bruner or Piaget, however, for Vygotsky semiotic mediation is critical to any description of development. Rather than depicting the child's progress as a series of staged steps of prior semiotic capacities (e.g., icons and indices prior to symbols and signs), Vygotsky claims that what develops are more differentiated functions of signs. For example, words, which are symbolic for adults, function first for children purely as indices. This indicatory or pointing function is never completely lost but is, rather, layered over with the more generalizing or categorizing function of true signs. In early adult-child communication, the word acts as an entry point, but only the label (and referent) is shared. The meaning relations are different, as Freud also noted in the child's use of *dead* (1900: 254). As the word is always a generalization – representing a type or class – use of a word leads the child into categorization even when the child is still using it as a token. On this view, then, regression would entail not so much thinking in images rather than words but thinking in words as images or using words in their earlier indicatory rather than their later semantic function. Words in dreams, and so forth, would thus represent tokens, and not types. As we can see, all three of these approaches have something to offer in understanding the concept of regression. (See figure 10.)

Bruner:	enactive → iconic → symbolic
Piaget:	signal → index → image → symbol → sign
Vygotsky:	word as image → word as index → word as category

Figure 10: The development of representational capacities: three views

In summary, dreams provided Freud with the material to build his royal road to an understanding of the unconscious as a repository of repressed knowledge. He took as axiomatic that knowledge is representational and sought to show the changes that those representations undergo due to repression, censorship, and so forth. His descriptions (along with his case studies, everyday pathologies, jokes, etc.) provide us with a remarkable account of the variety of representational forms that knowledge can take and of an alternate syntax to logical calculi, determining possible combinations and transformations of signs. Freud's work has more than justified Morris' claim that psychoanalysis among the psychologies has changed the way educated persons look at signs (1938: 38) and that "the field of psychopathology offers great opportunities for applications of, and contributions to, semiotic" (1938: 42).

In addition to a structural description, the important role Freud gave to the early childhood period in our lives raises questions about the development of (or diachronicity) of semiotic capacities. Since Freud's death, studies of representational intelligence in children have challenged some psychoanalytic conceptions of infant capacities: for example, Freud's hallucinatory wish fulfillment and the elaborate symbolization in infancy posited by Melanie Klein. An unresolved issue for psychoanalysis is whether the return of the repressed is as originally represented or as reconstructed by more fully developed representational capacities. This remains a critical question for any theory that hypothesizes a developmental arrest: will differences in kinds of illnesses – pre-Oedipal, Oedipal, borderline or narcissistic – be evident in representational differences of symptoms, dreams, and discourse?

4. Discourse

Through the study of pathology, psychoanalysis provides a window on the semiotic functioning of the human mind. Psychoanalysis also provides the best description we have of a psychic syntax – the types of psychological signs, the rules for their formation and expression – seen most clearly in descriptions of the dreamwork and case studies. This knowledge becomes a part of one's competence that is applied to the act of interpretation or reading of new signs in much the same way that our grammar is a finite set of rules enabling us to interpret even novel utterances. However, armed with only the grammar of the primary process and a book of symbolic equivalences (i.e., a dreambook) would be as ineffective as trying to understand an utterance with only a linguistic grammar and a dictionary. Syntax and the semantic equivalences of dictionary definitions provide only the skeleton for language in use. Meanings are created over time through dialogue with others and can, therefore, only be interpreted through negotiated discourses (Rommetveit 1974).

Psychoanalytic discourse is of a peculiar kind, negotiated under very specific conditions and circumstances. Freud had little to say about discourse directly. He did warn about the dangers of one-sided interpretation, of closing out the dreamer's role, for example, in the interpretation of dreams or their symbols

(1900: 353, 360;1901a: 684): "In the process of transforming a thought into a visual image a peculiar faculty is revealed by dreamers, and an analyst is rarely equal to following it with his guesses ... [one needs] the creator of these representations ... to explain their meaning" (1900: 361fn).

The critical move from the earlier talking cure to the importance of a transference neurosis is evidence that Freud felt the dialogic process had to be reengaged within the analysis for understanding to take place. He concluded that it is not sufficient for repressed material to escape repression by hooking up with verbal expression. That which is repressed – infantile wishes, unacceptable thoughts and ideas – must reappear in an peculiar discourse where: one participant has created signs whose meanings he does not know he knows and who thinks he wants to communicate but really doesn't; the other participant, armed with a knowledge of psychological signs and their syntax, tries to hear what isn't said and see what isn't shown. The one who really knows the meanings of the signs he has created (although he does not know he knows) is convinced that the other has this knowledge. How can this be so? The facile answer is that the other is an analyst, an expert who by definition has special knowledge. The real answer, however, is that an other (another other) was present and participated in the formation of the sign and that the analyst (as current other) represents those from past dialogues in the present one of analysis. The systematic regressions of transference neuroses provide insight and understanding precisely because they reenact patients' roles in dialogues from earlier periods in their lives with the analyst cast as significant others. If meanings were totally freed from their dialogic sources – what linguists call their "pragmatic contexts" – there could be no such phenomenon as transference.

Freud had little to say about the role of dialogue in the original creation of meanings, although some case materials are suggestive. For example, in exploring Little Hans' all important substitution of a horse for his father (mentioned above), Freud explains why a horse. It seems that Hans' father used to play at horses (play "horsey") with him. Similarly, the Wolfman's anxiety about wolves could be traced to a fairy-tale about seven little goats who were devoured by a wolf, just as his father in play jokingly used to threaten to gobble the Wolfman up (1926: 104). Herein one can glimpse the dialogic source of the symptom as sign.

Jacques Lacan (1977, 1978, 1968) has provided us with the best suggestion for the role of dialogue (or discourse) in the creation of the unconscious. I have suggested elsewhere (Litowitz n.d.) that on this topic Lacan's rereading of Freud is more radical than his focus on language in psychoanalysis, the role of which has been remarked on by other readers (Litowitz & Litowitz 1977; Forrester 1980; Edelson 1972). It is more radical because the internalization of the discourse of an other as constitutive of an individual unconscious is a conception more compatible with later object-relations theory than with Freud's original position of object-cathexis (Litowitz 1989; Greenberg & Mitchell 1983).[11]

If meanings are originally created in a dialogic process with significant others, then once again studies of development – here, developmental semantics and pragmatics – will be relevant to psychoanalysis. I have suggested elsewhere (Litowitz 1989) that developmental theories are available that are compatible with such an object-relations view of early psychological development. Psychoanalysis again can provide significant contributions to our understanding of the processes involved by means of the clinical evidence gathered from analytic discourses (Henriques et al. 1984).

In addition, because of the special constraints on analytic discourse, it provides a unique laboratory to discover the working of discourse in general. Careful examinations of how psychoanalytic discourse works from a semiotic perspective will surely add to our understanding of knowledge and the constitution of the self (e.g., Barratt 1984). Discourse is a part of pragmatics, the human use of signs in contexts of interactions, and questions of pragmatics (as opposed to semantics and syntax) are currently of great interest to linguists, philosophers, cognitive scientists, and others. Such theorists have been driven to pragmatics after discovering that the truth or falsehood of terms and propositions are indeterminate outside of the contexts of their use. The sanctity of decontextualized truth and falsehood has never been an issue for psychoanalysts. Psychoanalysis, therefore, could be in a position now to contribute as much to pragmatics as it has in the past to semantics and syntax.

Appendix: the role of semiotics in psychoanalysis

As is well known, Freud adapted the notion of energy as the force of movement in physical apparati (from mechanics) to the force that moves the psychic apparati. Whereas the laws of physics will explain the sources and destinies of energy as a force in the physical world, it remained for Freud to work out its vicissitudes in the psychical sphere. The power of this original metaphor is documented by the very fact and the myriad details of Freud's monumental *oeuvre*. The problems which attended the birth of this metaphor have been well documented (e.g., Gill 1976), vexing theorists who have tried to float psychoanalytic theory free from this foundation and place it on another (e.g., information theory, Peterfreund 1971). Linguistic theory and even semiotics have been discussed as possible new foundations (Edelson 1972; Lacan 1978; Rosen 1969; Martindale 1975; Mahoney & Singh 1975). The logic of such a choice is well motivated since, as we have seen, the data, its descriptions and explanations, that Freud addressed are sign phenomena, and often specifically verbal. The catch is that neither linguistic nor semiotic theory contains within it any element that could replace the function of energy in Freud's theory; that is, as a motivational source of intentionality. Linguistics can provide an understanding of how languages are structured and a list of functions that language can serve. Explorations of its subspecialties, such as semantics, syntactics and pragmatics, can offer interesting categories through which to view psychological phenomena. However, even if we hypothesize that linguistic structure is emblematic of mental functioning as a whole (as in Lacan's view of the unconscious as structured like a natural language) we still need to account for how any one individual moves through that structure; for example, why one thing is repressed and not another; how out of that structure compromises are formed.

While linguistics and semiotics cannot rescue psychoanalysis from its own metapsychological dilemmas, these disciplines can provide a new and unifying perspective on the actual data of psychoanalysis: the presentation of symptoms and their alleviation through therapeutic interpretation of their unconscious meaning. Thus, I disagree with those who believe that had Freud been aware of linguistic/semiotic theories he would have used these instead of hydraulics; I do think we would have had a more unified description of clinical material and that semiotics can now help us to raise some interesting questions about diagnosis and treatment.

Notes

1. One consequence was that a schism arose in semiotics between semiologists following de Saussure and semioticians of other schools. These differences have been much overestimated and are not of interest to our topic.
2. See Litowitz (n.d.) on Jacques Lacan's use of Saussurean semiology in psychoanalysis.
3. Much has been made of the importance of Peircean triadic relations that cannot be reduced to dyadic relations such as de Saussure's signifier-signified (Eco 1984). Nevertheless, it is the nature of these relations not just their number that is significant since others, e.g., Ogden and Richards (1962), also posit signification as triangular process but fail to avoid a positivist position.
4. Compare what Peirce attempted for signs with what Jakobson (Jakobson & Halle 1956) accomplished for phonology and what a structuralist semantics attempts for meanings (Lyons 1977).

5. I have given an example of a word. A picture or visual image is primarily interpreted as an icon but it too has indexical and symbolic representational potentials.
6. Although Freud later saw anxiety as arising from the ego, the issues of representation and substitution remain the same (1926: 161).
7. De Saussure also noted that "a particular word is like the center of a constellation: it is the point of convergence of an indefinite number of co-ordinated terms" (1959: 126).
8. See also the syntactic permutations in the dream of the botanical monograph (Litowitz 1977).
9. Freud adds: "Behind this childhood of the individual we are promised a picture of a phylogenetic childhood – a picture of the development of the human race" (1900: 548).
10. For Piaget, this constitutes primary symbolism. The special sense of Freudian symbols is secondary, i.e., a later addition.
11. Freud hinted at the possible continuation of a biological mother-foetus unit, wherein the mother satisfies all the foetus' needs with her own body, into a psychical object-relations dyad with the mother continuing to satisfy the infant's needs "though partly by other means" (1926: 138). He did not elaborate further nor discuss the role of dialogue.

References

Baer, Eugen

1974 "Understanding Lacan", in: Leo Goldberger & Victor H. Rosen (eds.), 473–544.

1982 "The medical symptom: phylogeny and ontogeny", *American Journal of Semiotics* 1 (3), 17–34.

Bailey, Richard W., Ladislav Matejka & Peter Steiner (eds.)

1980 *The sign: semiotics around the world.* Ann Arbor MI: Michigan Slavic Publications.

Bain, B. (ed.)

1983 *The sociogenesis of language and human conduct: a multidisciplinary book of readings.* New York: Plenum

Barratt, Barnaby B.

1984 *Psychic reality and psychoanalytic knowing.* Hillsdale NJ: The Analytic Press.

Breuer, Josef & Sigmund Freud
1893–95 *Studies on hysteria.* S.E. II. London: The Hogarth Press.
Bruner, Jerome
1973 "The growth of representational processes in childhood", in: *Beyond the information given.* New York: Norton, 313–324.
Bruss, Neal
1980 "The birth of psychoanalysis in semiotics, or of semiotics in psychoanalysis", in: Richard W. Bailey, Ladislav Matejka & Peter Steiner (eds.), 119–131.
Eco, Umberto
1984 *Semiotics and the philosophy of language.* Bloomington IN: Indiana University Press.
Edelson, Marshall
1972 "Language and dreams: *The interpretation of dreams* revisted", Psychoanalytic Study of the Child. 27, 203–282.
Field, Kay, Bertram Cohler & Glorye Woll (eds.)
1989 *Learning and education: psychoanalytic perspectives.* (Emotions and Behavior Monographs no. 6.) New York: International Universities Press.
Forrester, John
1980 *Language and the origins of psychoanalysis.* New York: Columbia University Press.
Freud, Sigmund
1885 "Report on my studies in Paris and Berlin", S.E. I, 1–15. London: The Hogarth Press.
1893 "Some points for a comparative study of oganic and hysterical motor paralyses", [1888–1893] S.E. I, 155–172. London: The Hogarth Press.
1895a *Project for a scientific psychology.* S.E. I, 281–397. London: The Hogarth Press.
1895b "On the grounds for detaching a particular syndrome from neurasthenia under the description 'anxiety neurosis'", S.E. III, 87–115. London: The Hogarth Press.
1896 "Further remarks on the neuro-psychoses of defence", S.E. III, 157–185. London: The Hogarth Press.
1898 "The psychical mechaism of forgetfulness", S.E. III, 287–297. London: The Hogarth Press.
1900 *The interpretation of dreams.* S.E. IV & V. London: The Hogarth Press.
1901a *On dreams.* S.E. V, 629-686. London: The Hogarth Press.
1901b *The psychopathology of everyday life.* S.E. VI. London: The Hogarth Press.

1905 "Fragment of an analysis of a case of hysteria", S.E. VII, 3–122. London: The Hogarth Press.

1911 "Psycho-analytic notes on an autobiographical account of a case of paranoia (dementia paranoides)", S.E. XII, 3–82. London: The Hogarth Press.

1913 "The claims of psycho-analysis to scientific interest", S.E. XIII, 163–190. London: The Hogarth Press.

1915 "The unconscious", S.E. XIV, 159-215. London: The Hogarth Press.

1916–17 *The introductory lectures on psycho-analysis*. S.E. XV & XVI. London: The Hogarth Press.

1917 "A metapsychological supplement to the theory of dreams", S.E. XIV, 217–235. London: The Hogarth Press.

1926 *Inhibitions, symptoms, and anxiety*. S.E. XX, 77–174. London: The Hogarth Press.

Gill, Merton M.

1976 "Metapsychology is not psychology", in: Merton M. Gill & Philip S. Holzman (eds.), 71–105.

Gill, Merton M. & Philip S. Holzman (eds.)

1976 *Psychology versus metapsychology*. Psychological Issues IX no. 4. New York: International Universities Press.

Goldberg, Arnold (ed.)

1983 *The future of psychoanalysis*. New York: International Universities Press.

Goldberger, Leo & Victor H. Rosen (eds.)

1974 *Psychoanalysis and contemporary science*. Vol. 3. New York: International Universities Press.

Greenberg, Jay R. & Stephen A. Mitchell

1983 *Object relations in psychoanalytic theory*. Cambridge, MA: Harvard University Press.

Henriques, Julian, Wendy Hollway, Cathy Urwin, Couze Venn & Valerie Walkerdine.

1984 *Changing the subject: psychology, social regulation & subjectivity*. London: Methuen.

Jakobson, Roman & Morris Halle

1956 *Fundamentals of language*. The Hague: Mouton

Lacan, Jacques

1968 *The language of the self: the function of language in psychoanalysis*. (Translated with notes and commentary by Anthony Wilden.) Baltimore MD: John Hopkin Press.

1977 *Écrits*. New York: Norton.
1978 The four fundamental concepts of psycho-analysis. New York: Norton.

Litowitz, Bonnie E.
1977 "Individual and shared meaning", *Papers in Linguistics* 10 (3–4), 341–373. (Edmonton, Canada: Linguistic Research.)
1978 "On overdetermination", in: Joseph H. Smith (ed.), 355–394.
1989 "Patterns of internalization", in: Kay Field, Bertram Cohler & Glorye Woll (eds.), 305–328.
n.d. "A linguist looks at Lacan".[Unpublished manuscript.]

Litowitz, Bonnie E. & Norman S. Litowitz
1977 "The influence of linguistic theory on psychoanalysis: a critical historical survey", *International Review of Psycho-analysis* 4, 419–448.
1983 "Development of verbal self-expression", in: Arnold Goldberg (ed.), 397–427.

Lyons, John
1977 *Semantics*. Vol. 1. Cambridge: Cambridge University Press.

Mahony, Patrick & Rajendra Singh
1975 "*The interpretation of dreams*, semiology and Chomskian linguistics: a radical critique", *Psychoanalytic Study of the Child* 30, 221–241.

Martindale, Colin
1975 "The grammar of altered states of consciousness: a semiotic reinterpretation of aspect of psychoanalytic theory", in: Donald P. Spence (ed.), 331–354.

Morris, Charles
1938 "Foundations of the theory of science", *Foundations of the unity of science*. Vols. 1–2. Chicago IL: University of Chicago Press.

Mueller-Vollmer, K.
1986 "Thinking and speaking: Heider, Humboldt and French semiotics", paper presented at Heider Conference, Monterey, California, November 1985, revised 1986. [To be published as part of conference proceedings.]

Neisser, Uriel
1967 *Cognitive psychology*. New York: Appleton Century-Crofts.

Ogden, C.K. & I.A. Richards
1962 *The meaning of meaning*. New York: Harcourt, Brace & World.

Peirce, Charles Sanders
1931–58 *Collected papers I-VIII*. (Edited by C. Hartshorne, P. Weiss & A. Burks) Cambridge MA: Harvard University Press.

1955 *Philosophical writings of Peirce*. (Selected & edited by Justus Buchler.) New York: Dover Publications.

Pelc, Jerzy
1981 "Theoretical foundations of semiotics", *American Journal of Semiotics* 1 (1–2), 15–45.

Peterfreud, Emanuel
1971 *Information, systems, and psychoanalysis: an evolutionary biological approach to psychoanalytic theory*. Psychological Issues VII nos. 1/2. New York: International Universities Press.

Piaget, Jean
1962 *Play, dreams, and imitation*. New York: Norton.

Rommetveit, Ragnar
1974 *On message structure*. New York: John Wiley.

Rosen, Victor H.
1969 "Sign phenomena and their relationship to unconscious meaning", *International Journal of Psycho-analysis* 50, 197–207.

Saussure, Ferdinand de
1959 *Course in general linguistics*. New York: Philosophical Library.

Schimek, Jean
1974 "The parapraxis specimen of psychoanalysis", in: Leo Goldberger & Victor H. Rosen (eds.), 210–130.

Smith, Joseph H. (ed.)
1978 *Psychiatry and the humanities*. Vol. 3. New Haven CT: Yale University Press.

Spence, Donald P. (ed.)
1975 *Psychoanalysis and contemporary science*. Vol. 4. New York: International Universities Press.

Vygotsky, Lev S.
1962 Thought and language. Cambridge MA: MIT Press.
1978 *Mind in society: the development of higher psychological processes*. (Edited by Michael Cole, Vera John-Steiner, Sylvia Scribner & Ellen Souberman.) Cambridge MA: Harvard University Press.

Wertsch, James
1983 "The role of semiosis in L.S. Vygotsky's theory of human cognition", in: B. Bain (ed.), 17–31.

Wilden, Anthony
1972 *System and structure*. London: Tavistock Publications.

Psychoanalysis without foundations

Arnold Goldberg

Introduction

A case is presented in a clinical seminar. Many questions are asked since the presenter has necessarily fashioned the content of the case in order to make certain issues more prominent, and, in doing so, has omitted material felt by him to be less cogent. The questioners feel differently about the comparative import of the issues with some stressing some points, while others concentrate elsewhere. At various points in the presentation it seems than an essentially well meaning listener can weave an explanation of the case that is clear, coherent and telling. Yet at other moments, the same can be said of another listener whose set of ideas seem equally plausible and convincing, yet somewhat at odds with the first. Almost anyone seems capable of fashioning some sort of meaning out of the case, although one or two may sound more persuasive than others. But the sense of conviction, that may or may not arrive, yields no certain clue as to whether it comes from the logic of the argument, the vigor of the deliverer or one's personal preconceptions as to what to favor.

As in any sort of disagreement an effort is made to move forth from certain agreed upon facts or notions, and to determine if one can argue over and resolve the points of divergence. For instance, a patient is reported as saying something, and surely there is no disagreement over the uttered words. Perhaps one member of the audience even takes issue here and wonders about the tone and feelings carried by the sentence as well as what was left unsaid. And another listener claims that no sentence can be lifted out of context, since it stands embedded in a dialogue with the analyst and linked to everything said before. Alas, it seems, that we may never get started on the path of understanding.

The group may splinter into clusters of general agreement, or else an effort is begun to see if a prerequisite for discussion is some form of declared affiliation: something like belonging to a league of like believers who need not argue over each and every word. Thus the larger group may reform into islands of separate thought or else into a network of wonder and confusion which can only hope ultimately to coalesce into a coherent whole. It may be said that the varying conceptualizations of the case are but redescriptions of the material using different vocabularies to say things in a different way. But the speakers would not agree that they are saying the same thing, since at some point they feel that their rendition is more authentic or closer to the truth. Indeed, this is what lies behind each narrative: a conviction of something more fundamental and more real. It is as if somewhere there lies a point of uniform and universal agreement; a place where the disagreement ceases and consensus is achieved. All of our conferences seem to yearn for such a place. But this problem is not that of psychiatric and/or psychoanalytic conferences alone. It is in its own way, a part of every other discipline's quest for knowledge: the thirst for foundation and certainty.

1. Philosophic background

Best known in the search for foundations is the famous *cognito ergo sum* of Rene Descartes, the philosopher who claimed that one could doubt everything save one's own existence. Skeptics have since undermined even that noted resting place (Stroud 1984), but that effort inevitably seems to lead to what Richard Bernstein calls the Cartesian anxiety: "Either there is some support for our being, a fixed foundation for our knowledge, or we cannot escape the forces of darkness that envelop us with madness, with intellectual and moral chaos" (1986: 10–11).

The most eminent classical foundationalist of this century, C.J. Lewis, held that "unless something is certain, nothing else is even probable" (1952: 168). The argument over such foundations is carried on within philosophical circles between those who claim that certainly what we observe is true or real (Dancy 1985:101), and those who believe that there are many versions of the world, and thus there is no one right way of describing it (Goodman & Elgin 1987); i.e., every rendition is a redescription with none more right than another.

The arguments for and against declaring what is sensed or observed to be true is most apparent and also most cogent outside of psychology, in the so-called natural sciences. There it is said that people can and should agree on the existence of things, on the nature of numbers, on visible behavior, etc. Even here, however, this position has been challenged, since now it is felt that, to paraphrase Kuhn, there is no neutral algorithm for theory-choice, no systematic decision process which, properly applied, must lead each individual in the group to the same decision (1970). But it is even more so the case in the effort to circumscribe individual intentions, beliefs and meanings that there is a lack of consensus or any easy or systematic way that people can be shown to agree. Between the insistence on the hard facts of real things and the equal resoluteness on the indeterminacy of personal feelings, there lies within psychoanalysis that large space for disagreement about the nature of what we know for sure that one finds in all of science. We may certainly come to agreement more readily about the time of day than about how you or I may feel about something.

2. Psychoanalytic background

The psychoanalyst, like all scientists, starts with shared beliefs. Samuel Guttman (1985) lists for us the fundamental tenets of psychoanalysis as: the recognition of the existence of unconscious mental processes; the mechanism of repression; infantile sexuality and the Oedipus complex, and their importance for psychic life, particularly for psychopathology; and at other times, as a recognition of phenomena of transference and resistance as a frame of reference in analysis. Guttman says that proponents of deviant theories or those that depart from the tenets have questioned the competence of others and have made frontal attacks upon the others' personalities. In an almost blinding sleight of hand maneuver, Guttman tells us that the true test of a deviant theory is the incongruity between the aspiration and the creative power of the deviant. Thus his particular frontal attack on the personality of the creative individual consists in the fact that individuals fall short of the wish to be creative in forging a new theory, i.e., they were disappointing in their results. They aimed too high.

If one considers the listed tenets of Guttman in turn, then a considerable amount of disagreement or debate may be generated by each of them. (1) The existence of unconscious mental phenomena: though this may be a hallmark of psychoanalysis, it suffers from the lack of clarity of definition. For Lacan, the unconscious is structured like a language and is a repository of signifiers, while for others it contains memories, and for still others, universal forms of fantasies. Jung insisted on a phylogenetic unconscious domain. Melanie Klein opted for an early elaboration of destructive fantasies; and recently Schimek (1975) stated that the concept of unconscious representation must be abandoned entirely. We agree on the unconscious but seemingly cannot circumscribe its makeup. (2) The mechanism of repression: there is no doubt that repression was considered central to Freud's theory of neurosogenesis. Time has certainly eroded that centrality with the elaboration of other defense mechanisms, with some scholars (Basch 1983) claiming that disavowal or denial hold equal prominence to repression. As developmental issues began to dominate analytic thinking, considerations of developmental arrest called for reformulations of psychopathology that seemed not to include repression as primary (Stolorow & Brandchaft 1987). As a consequence, repression becomes less central or even dismissed. (3) Infantile sexuality and the Oedipus complex, and their importance for psychic life: once again the departure from Freud is evident in these concepts with some authors dismissing Oedipal material as primary and others downplaying the role of infantile sexuality. With Melanie Klein's work, aggressive issues began to dominate and pre-Oedipal phenomena were noted by Ernest Jones in his Freud biography to have been neglected by his mentor. Winnicott (1965) felt that the whole world of infancy was poorly appreciated by Freud. Thus the significance of infantile sexuality and the Oedipus complex become diminished. (4) Transference and resistance: Bird (1972) tells us that there are as many imputations of significance to transference as there are analysts. The familial transferences of Freud have been expanded to narcissistic ones; the neurotic ones have been expanded to the psychotic. The concept of resistance is equally debated, discussed, dissected, and dismissed.

More important than all of the ferment of disagreement over all of these basic concepts is the larger concern that, although they may be a part of psychoanalysis, even as a group they are certainly not equivalent to psychoanalysis. Transference and resistance are universal phenomena and are now well incorporated into all forms of psychotherapy as well as in many studies of human behavior. The unconscious, repression, the Oedipus complex are no strangers to any student of the social sciences, and they all seem to owe an allegiance to psychoanalysis without being peculiar to it. Indeed, most psychotherapists would say these are all basic tenets of their own field, which is not psychoanalysis *per se*. If one carefully examines any single one of the concepts, there is no doubt there are points in their application where an analyst would say that the term is no longer that of strict psychoanalysis. One might, for instance, see the evidence of resistance in some personal encounter without in any way saying this constituted a psychoanalysis. Not the single tenet nor the sum of the tenets makes for the field. No matter how much agreement would be reached in these concepts, the disagreements would be severe, and the claim to uniqueness would be lost. There seems no easy way to say this idea or these concepts are the rock bottom of psychoanalysis. They do not belong uniquely to psychoanalysis, nor do they define it.

If we return to the case conference, we can listen to varied explanations of the case which may utilize some or all of these basic tenets with an admixture of others. Seemingly each listener operates with some framework of acceptable ideas in mind. If, for instance, a speaker would invoke extrasensory perception as an explanatory vehicle, there would be a clear exception taken by the audience claiming that a boundary has been overstepped. Guttman (1985) uses the example of Eysenck as someone who is clearly outside the fold, since his ideas can be considered nonanalytic or antianalytic. He cites Binswanger as one psychoanalyst who embraced the existential school of psychiatry but could not be considered as deviant, since he made no claim of being a creator of a new psychology. Thus it may come about that the personal claim of the theorist becomes a determiner of deviance. And, since Guttman insists that the claim must be substantiated as worthy of a "creator of the first rank", then we must wait until he or someone else has properly evaluated that claim. As in many similar efforts at creativity, at times a wider net is cast to build a case; i.e., we reach outside of psychoanalysis *per se* both for new ideas and for firmer bedrock.

Not every field seems so eager to seek such outside support for its data. The natural sciences appear to operate within a set of rules which enable agreement; i.e., either the experiment yields helium or it does not. Only a historical survey of these sciences reveals the gradual erosion and re-definition of their rules, procedures and definitions. But the problem is much more acute in psychoanalysis which seemingly allows everyone in the conference to be on equal footing. The way to win the day seems more and more to demand a drastic re-description: a whole new vocabulary. And this is best achieved by carving out a new area for inquiry. We shall look at two.

3. Infant observation

Going outside of the analytic setting to validate what goes on inside is said by some (Grünbaum 1984) to be absolutely necessary. Psychoanalysts must become grounded on firmer terrain than the shared constructs of patient and analyst. The recent investigation of infant behavior is one such effort, and it has sparked a recrudescence of modifications of psychoanalytic theory that are aimed at conforming to the new findings of this field of infant observation. It is felt that the careful study of infancy can lend a basis to adult psychology, one that is otherwise only inferred or assumed from the study of adults. The results of these infant observations are felt to stand on firmer ground than some of the ideas developed in analytic studies of adults. For example, the attribution of imagining or reflecting upon a memory in an infant under eighteen months of age flies in the face of Piaget's studies on evocative memory (Piaget & Inhelder 1969). Thus one needs to alter or modify a theory which demands that infantile hallucination explains the behavior of an infant. We embark on a road of a new sort of factual information which alters the inferred material. So, too, does Basch say that attributing the capacity to a newborn infant of imitating the face of an adult is in error, since the skills necessary for imitation are simply not present in a newborn (1988: 75). There is a certain sense of sureness lent to the new knowledge about infancy that seems more able to ground the data that analysts may use. Thus the new grounding may allow us to reshape or alter the basic tenets and even to totally discard them. At last, we may know for sure.

Lichtenberg (1983) tells us that "experience" is contained in his hypotheses about infancy, and that this is a necessarily speculative area. Our certainty starts to unravel. Stern states that "the discoveries of developmental psychology are dazzling, but they seem doomed to remain clinically sterile unless one is willing to make *inferential leaps* about what they may mean for the *subjective life* of the infant" (1985: 5). [Emphasis added] The work of Lichtenberg and Stern speaks of the subjective states of an infant, all of which are necessarily and perhaps regrettably inferred by the researcher since these infants only betray their feelings; they do not speak of them. Soon there emerges a sobering quality to the excitement of these new findings as we learn that our own contributions to the mix seem inevitably to yield a new recipe. We do not all share speculations or inferential leaps, until and unless we have earlier shared some other common ground. The observations of infants become subject to the same erosive process as did the basic tenets of psychoanalysis. And here again, we falter and try to go further or deeper. The observations of infants do not prove or disprove anything but rather become additional factors limiting analytic findings; the kind of limiting factors that any science must consider. They may be new descriptions, but we wonder if they are improved descriptions.

4. Neurology

Neurology or neurophysiology may be the answer. We argue over the existence of (say) multiple personality disorder, and we are shown a positron emission tomography (PET) scan of patients who have different emergent personalities. The one personality named John is clearly different on the readout from the one named George, and so the argument may be at an end. Proof lies before us in a perception that can be shared by an unlimited number of observers. This is no longer a matter of opinion but has gained the status of a fact.

In another example psychodynamic and psychoanalytic ideas about the characterological state of shyness are presented as deriving from some defensive operations against either exhibitionism or aggression. But then some genetic studies show that there is a strong familial tendency to the existence of shyness, and soon after there seems to emerge some neuroanatomical and biochemical underpinnings to the tenets of shyness that need have little to do with the psychodynamic explanations offered for the development of this sort of personality. And once again the psychological stance seems to give way to the neurological. Of course we may hear that the brain acting differently in supposedly different personalities is just evidence of something. Although that something is psychological, need it be translated into truly distinct and different persons residing in one mind; or, is that an unwarranted inference? And so, too, we may hear the protest that shyness still maintains its psychological significance though underpinned by biological evidence. One type of evidence need not supersede the other, but our bent is to give in to the neurology, to the hard facts of science.

Freud felt that ultimately all psychological issues would be found to have their basis in some sort of neuroanatomical or neurohormonal comprehension. Many others have shared this posture that effectively makes of psychology a temporary waystation or resting place to the true answers of human behavior which must ultimately be in the brain. There is even a philosophical school of thought called eliminative materialism which takes as its main thesis the position that the findings in neurology, including all the subspecialties with the neuro- prefix, will, over time, manage to correct and then finally eliminate the psychological. On this view, what passes for psychology is not really a scientific enterprise but is really something called folk psychology. Take, for example, any known and agreed upon psychological trait such as shyness or stinginess or compulsiveness. These can be defined in some behavioristic manner just like the perception of colors or odors may be. Now, if we can determine with some accuracy just what the neurological underpinnings to these bits of psychology may be, we may be able to declare if they are valid states, and then we may exchange these forms of psychology for neurology. Thus, if the same neurons are involved in both the traits of state a and state b , then we may learn that our division into two states was erroneous and unnecessary. Not only that, but the more proper and correct view of these states is seen to be the neuronal configuration. We can then dispense with the cumbersome field of psychology and replace it with a scientific neurology.

The conclusion follows that one day all beliefs and desires will be seen as essentially unscientific statements that can be traced to their neurological source and ultimately eliminated, i.e., as far as scientists are concerned. Now this is obviously an oversimplification, and some philosophers as well as neurologists scoff at that ultimate possibility. But it does point to the thesis that the ground of psychology lies in the brain and its functioning, and that this claims priority in the adjudicating of a foundation.

The response to this stance asks if it is possible to eliminate the psychological. If two distinct states are declared to be but one, we would not necessarily need to accept this. Indeed, the facts are that our psychology really is primary, and it directs our neurological searches. We know our beliefs and desires as facts, and we cannot be persuaded to abandon them by claims from another discipline. Even our evaluation of shyness as a defense against exhibitionism can claim the same status of certainty as can the determination of a brain area responsible for its existence. There is no inherent supremacy of neurology save as psychology shrinks away from its own claims of knowing. Rather it is the haunting conviction that we do not seem capable of certainty that allows psychoanalysis to too easily retreat before the counterclaims of other disciplines. The neurologists hold arms together in a solid phalanx of sureness shown by the PET scan or electroencephalography (EEG) or brain section, and the analyst usually retreats before them. He does so primarily by adopting the test of certainty used by those other scientists.

To some extent every science may give way before another which lays claim to giving causal explanations to its data. Thus much social behavior is made clear by way of psychoanalytic insights, just as physics can be employed to give the crucial causal explanations to chemistry. Disciplines draw their boundaries based on tools as well as on the content of the field. Once defined, the discipline can stay within its fences or else venture out with the known risk of redefinition and/or the creation of a new discipline as in the example of physical chemistry serving to bridge the two areas. Such efforts have been suggested for psychoanalysis which has been urged to adopt information theory (Peterfreund 1971) or systems theory or communication theory to enable it to obliterate the agreed upon boundary. It is said that information theory, for example, will unite neurophysiology and psychiatry and allow us to build a floor under the floating set of ideas that serve analysis (Basch 1988).

One response to such suggestions for unity is that of insisting that the adoption of nonanalytic theories (i.e., theories without analytic data) robs us of the richness of the consulting room and thus takes us away from the true study of analysis. Rather, psychoanalysis need only stay within its realm of inquiry and rely only on the elements of coherence and fittedness to be capable of the claim of validity. Heinz Kohut, for instance, insisted that the field of psychoanalysis was defined by its method: empathy. Therefore only the data obtained by empathy belonged to the field and only it could be used to validate the field. Infant research, neurology and the rest of biology, etc. were of interest only as they allowed one's empathy to expand and to push further into the realm of data gathering. But these other sources did not explain anything in analysis; they dealt with different material entirely. In a way it is a scandal in psychoanalysis that there seems to be so little confidence in its methods and its data. Our clinical seminar participants (mentioned at the start of my paper), in truth, do not behave as do rival chemists studying a single experiment, but more as rival experimenters gathering different data. They listen to different parts, emphasize different elements, and form different conclusions. Everyone seems qualified to put things together in his or her own way given the limiting factors that serve as baseline, i.e., those agreed upon rules such as no ESP, etc. The issues offered to us in infant observation and neurology help us to draw the boundaries, but the content must and should fundamentally be the data of analysis. Essentially what happens in the conference is the practice of understanding the patient. One has a right to challenge whether a particular description of the patient yields a picture that does contribute to understanding or else stops that pursuit by a claim of a different sort; i.e., it is really only a certain sort of brain reaction.

As one ponders over the very obvious distinction between the way analysts operate, versus the observations made in infant research and neurophysiology, it seems to be true that a different sort of knowledge gathering is at work: that of understanding another person. This lays claim to a unique way of knowing, and perhaps the longed for foundations lie in that direction.

5. Understanding and explanation

Some years ago I was participating as an examiner for the boards in psychiatry. One applicant, who was primarily a neurologist but wanted to have an expertise in psychiatry, had just finished an interview with a patient, someone who had a variety of behavior disorders including that of exposing himself to women. The applicant suffered not only from a limitation in his knowledge but also had difficulty with the English language. He stumbled badly over his presentation to me of the interview, not only because of his anxiety, but also because he seemed quite lost in his grasp of the patient. After a few leading questions he seemed to be getting on the track about the patient and suddenly with a sense of enlightenment and a great deal of vigor pronounced: "The man is an exhibitionist!" The applicant seemed relieved and pleased with his newfound understanding of the case. But then he was pushed further beyond this conclusion with a question asking just why this was the case; i.e., "Why is he an exhibitionist?" The applicant became startled and clearly forlorn and turned to the questioner with arms out and palms up saying, "But how should I know?"

Essentially this man claimed understanding but without explanation. Those two words, explanation and understanding, have haunted psychoanalysis for many years. Heinz Hartmann (1964) reviewed the concepts some time ago and claimed that understanding alone is never sufficient, that it was not to be considered to be *the* method of psychology but rather that psychoanalysis is an explanatory psychology which is empirically verifiable, i.e., grounded in fact. One needs at the outset to clarify these two words, since we can all claim to understand something that is explained to us as well as (occasionally) to be able to explain something that is understood. Kohut (1984) claimed that depth psychology explained what is first understood and so does both, and thus is basically a psychology of understanding. To that last point we would all, including Hartmann, agree: we understand both the rational meaning of communication as well as the motives behind it. But for Hartmann that is only the beginning, and it by no means distinguishes psychoanalysis, which has its special status by way of its explanations. And here is where Kohut fails us, albeit in a different way than does Hartmann. The latter tells us that understanding refers to the connections of meaning structures, while explanation refers to causal relationships based upon instinctual processes. For Hartmann the natural science status of psychoanalysis lies in its biological base; specifically, in the theory of drives. For Kohut, explanation lies within the narrative story of the patient, and so he would "explain" a patient's anger as being directed toward the analyst's absence and derived from the empathic failure, i.e., absence of the parental function. Indeed these are two sorts of explanation, and we soon shall see that many things can and do serve as explanations (Spence 1986).

We explain a patient's anger at his wife as really being directed at the analyst. We explain the anger toward the analyst as really being meant for the mother. We explain the anger at the mother as a product of an aggressive drive and/or an injury to the self. We explain the aggression as due to a particular form of child rearing, perhaps in combination with some biological givens. We explain the child rearing as either innate or cultural and beneath that there lies a consideration of the neuronal pathways for aggression and/or the biochemical substrates (remember the shy child). At any point in this sequence we may feel completely satisfied with the explanation. At all points we may understand the patient based on any one or all of the explanations. And again at any point we may feel that we have reached bedrock, that our explanation(s) offer(s) a foundation for our comprehension and that we need go no further. But, sadly, at any point we may be wrong. For if we trace in the opposite direction the sequence of causality from the biochemistry to the mental strife, we can see that we may have spun a story that has credibility but certainly lies far away from certainty. We know that, for instance, development may take many forms and many paths, and retrospective analysis deals with enormous complexities, while progressive study offers innumerable possibilities. Every step to put a floor under our conceptulization allows us a temporary pause of relief only to watch it inevitably disappear as alternatives let themselves be heard.

Let us recapitulate the problem. At the very first level there is a two-party agreement between patient and analyst as to what is to be accepted as real or true or factual. The analyst understands the patient's meanings and a story begins to take form. This story or narrative is bounded by the context of treatment (Schafer 1975) and, of course, is one of many that could be constructed. Spence is clearly unhappy at stopping here and says, "... narrative coherence is needed to make the case report more accessible ... but must not be used to provide an explanation of events in the case; this function is now taken over by attempts to relate specific events to more general classes and the classes, in turn, to theoretical propositions" (1975: 16). Thus he pleads for a public airing of case reports to extend the claim of credibility beyond that of the cloistered pair that form the narrative. Hartmann and others would probably say that this, too, rests on an understanding of the case, albeit by people who share a common language, but explanation must go beyond this to determine the causal factors involved, ones that are empirically justified. The developmentalist would argue that the empirical justification of the story, i.e., the causal factors, can and do derive from our knowledge of development gathered outside of the consulting room. Thus no true or reliable story can be constructed that does not conform to normal development and its problems; and ultimately we may have a compendium of allowable stories to constrain the overly liberal weaving of events knitted by some analysts. The neurologist would say that it is perfectly fine to construct such studies, but their fate is uncertain since ultimately they will be eliminated by proper brain studies, and only then can we and should we be satisfied. It is unnecessary for us to go beyond the neurologist at this point, but it should be clear that one may go on to chemistry and physics and beyond. There is no end point presently in sight.

Of course, it should be clear that these jumps are dictated by theoretical postures and involve different vocabularies, different methods of data gathering and sometimes wholly different forms of facts or data. It is also true that the discourse in one realm is not easily, and sometimes not ever, translatable to another. On some occasions a new theory obliterates distinctions, but it may also be true that there are unbridgeable gaps. For example, some feel that the study of molecular genetics will not ever explain how organisms come into being but will remain at the level of correlation, e.g., between deoxyribonucleic acid (DNA) and phenotype. But with all of these qualifications we can draw a sort of continuum with a series of resting places, some of which will be satisfactory for some individuals while none will satisfy everyone. At this point choice among foundations seems to become but a matter of choice or even of taste.

Understanding is a necessary and significant part of psychoanalytic knowledge, but people may understand a case in a different manner. We listen to each case with a particular theory in mind just as each case is presented with a particular theory in mind. Once understood we may choose to explain the case with the same set of theoretical principles with which we listened or even with a new set. The latter activity aims at grounding the understanding, transforming it into what is usually a causal sequence that makes sense in a different way than the understanding did. Since understanding *per se* is such a prominent component of psychoanalysis, its study is a proper area of focus. Along with this effort there is the corollary one of interpretation, since that activity for some is equivalent to understanding. However, as Habermas says: "... as soon as observed modes of behavior have to be interpreted ..., the conditions are no longer given independently of the interpretation of the actor himself. Interpretive schema are interposed between the stimulus and the responding behavior, and they must be uncovered, because they perform the world view as well as the needs of the actor" (1988: 101). We understand through our knowing about other people's viewpoints, i.e., their interpretations, and we further impose our interpretations upon the process. This connection between subject and object is what Apel calls "an interpretive rediscovery of one's self in the other" (1984: 36) and leads us into another vexing problem in psychoanalysis: the science of interpretation, or hermeneutics.

6. Hermeneutics

There can be no doubt that psychoanalysis deals with hermeneutics. Some analysts, however, think that that is an unfortunate state of affairs because, they are convinced, hermeneutical investigations make for wild and wooly speculations that just further undermine the empirical status of their field and lead even more to a standard-less climate of "anything goes". To fully explore the role of hermeneutics would require an independent exposition. For the purpose of the present discussion, two opposing viewpoints championed by two scholars, Hirsch and Gadamer, may help to focus us on the issue of standards.

Hans-Georg Gadamer published *Truth and method* in 1960 and focused philosophic attention on hermeneutics. His concern was to overcome the wish to feel that we can develop "objective" knowledge of phenomena. For Gadamer understanding is primarily an effort to come to understanding with others. Such an understanding is embedded in history and arises along with our prejudices and our subjectivity. We understand both truths and intentions: the first has to do with knowledge like geometry; while the second involves motives of other persons (Warnke 1987).

E.D. Hirsch has been cited by Rubovitz-Seitz (1986) as author of a solution to the problem of unlimited interpretations. Hirsch says that texts mean what the author intends, and Rubovitz-Seitz follows this general principle in pursuing the meaning of patients' productions. Hirsch feels that one can unearth what an author (and from this point on we will be free to substitute "patient") means by such hermeneutic methods as guesses, comparisons and reexperiences. In this manner one shares a meaning with the patient. Although Hirsch would endorse the view that in reading one enters a new domain, he would disagree that this means that one now operates under new rules or standards. Interpretation still depends upon the author's intentions.

Gadamer feels that sharing involves more than sharing meaning; rather, it involves the construction of a shared language. Thus meaning cannot be attributed to either writer or reader (patient or analyst); it is not one person's possession but becomes a common view of the two participants. For Gadamer, participants in reading, writing and speaking are the creators of meaning. He makes this point in order to explain the fact that works of art can be different each time they are encountered, even though they remain self-identical.

For Hirsch a work of art is determinate and is not dependent on the audience. He claims that one can still try to determine the author's intention even if viewed or read by different audiences. One could, in disagreement with Hirsch, argue that authors do not or need not know their intentions, but Gadamer goes further than this. He claims that every achievement of understanding is relative to the audience that perceives it and so involves participation. In this way, we are returned to the possibility that interpretation is arbitrary, since everyone perceives in the context of his or her own situation.

To answer the accusation that asking us to ascertain "the truth of the object" invites us to substitute our prejudice for another's, Gadamer states that all interpretation is prejudice. One cannot appeal to an "objective" basis for understanding, such as an author's intentions, the scientific method, or even the perspective of God. Rather we grant what he calls "normative authority" to the object and apply it so that it makes sense for our situation. This resolution of the tension between the prejudices of one's own truth claims and those of another is resolved in the model of a Socratic dialogue (Warnke 1987: 101). This consensus, which Gadamer calls a "fusion of horizons", achieves a synthesis of two separate positions and represents a new, third view. Thus truth is never final or exhaustive, and even though understanding is a comprehension of meaning, the meanings themselves can also change.

As Warnke says: "For hermeneutic understanding it follows that we are not limited to the premises of our tradition but rather continually revise them in the encounters with and discussions we have of them" (1987: 170). Now this view creates a radically different perspective for our clinical seminar example. We do not all independently observe a fixed entity but rather successively construct one. A radical shift occurs when we allow our participants the freedom to bring a set of beliefs or prejudices to the meeting and thus yield a variety of syntheses.

7. Conclusion

Perhaps our case seminar had the wrong goal in mind. Perhaps it should not have been designed so much to understand the patient as to understand and remake ourselves. To do so one must listen to each and every participant who seemingly has the truth in hand, as though in a conversation which may end either in agreement or disagreement, but which may also lead to a new synthesis. If we incorporate all the findings of all the bedrock truths of every participant, then we embark on a spiral of a new complete understanding, of a never certain set of truths. Thus we are keeping the conversation going (Rorty 1989). Foundations end the conversation, since nothing more need be said. Self-evident truths solve things, once and for all. But why should psychoanalysis be able to enjoy that sort of resolution any more than any science can be said to be capable of final solutions?

In this paper I have addressed the position of psychoanalysis among the other sciences, the discussions that go on within the field of psychoanalysis, and the content of the analytic situation; and it may be a mistake to lump them all together as forms of conversation and/or as non-foundational pursuits. On the other hand, they do indeed share a common activity: the gathering up of knowledge. Viewed in this way, legitimate next questions might be: is there some inherent non-foundational position to anything and everything we do and say; does anything stand for anything or is it all up for grabs; are foundations ever outside our grasp; and, if so, how does one ever agree to agree?

Richard Rorty (1989) makes a contrast for us between persons he calls "ironists" and those who are "commonsensical". He tells us that everyone has a vocabulary to fit their view of the world. Ironists are those who have continuing doubts about their vocabulary, who realize that arguments phrased in that vocabulary can neither confirm nor dissolve these doubts, and finally who do not think their vocabulary is closer to reality than others. They realize that anything can be made to look good or bad by being redescribed; they are thus always aware of the contingency and fragility of their words and their selves. Common sense, on the other hand, takes for granted that the inherited vocabulary provides a picture of knowledge as a relation between human beings and "reality". Such persons believe the world is there, and it is our duty to discover it; "redescription" is to be avoided. Such a position thinks that getting things right is to grasp the "real essence", to obtain the truth. In contrast, the ironist says right means 'suitable for those who speak as we do', who share our vocabularies.

Mankind needs heroes, addictions and rules: they all bring us together; resolve our doubts; steer us against our feelings of fragility; and convince us that we are closer to reality. They should and do make sense of things and should and do resolve uncertainty. They remove the haunting fear that we may be constructing a set of fairy tales for explanation. They allow us to stand foursquare with the hard scientists who can replicate data and know things that can stand up to time and trial. The problem is that they themselves may well be a fairy tale of our own making. It is not only because these constraints are imprisoning that we are forced to question them; they are unlikely to be other than just one way of talking about things (as the ironist claims everything really is). Is it possible that we have allowed ourselves to be convinced of the so-called commonsense way of the world, and have so become prisoners of our own making? Language is a prisonhouse and the assumption of foundations is another. Doing without certainty is liberating, and there is no greater liberation than the free use of language. Psychoanalysis would do well to embrace and share this freedom.

References

Apel, K.O.
1984 *Understanding and explanation.* (Translated by Georgia Warnke.) Cambridge MA: MIT Press.
Basch, Michael F.
1983 "The perception of reality and the disavowal of meaning", *The Annual of Psychoanalysis* 11, 125–134. New York: International Universities Press.
1988 *Understanding psychotherapy.* New York: Basic Books.
Bernstein, Richard J.
1986 *Philosophical profiles.* Philadelphia PA: University of Pennsylvania Press.
Bird, Brian
1972 "Notes on transference: universal phenomenon and hardest part of analysis", *Journal of the American Psychoanalytic Association* 20 (2), 267–301.
Dancy, J.
1985 *Introduction to contemporary epistemology.* New York: Basil Blackwell.
Goodman, N. & C. Elgin
1987 *Reconceptions in philosophy and other arts and sciences.* London: Routledge.
Grünbaum, Adolf
1984 *The foundations of psychoanalysis: a philosophical critique.* Berkeley CA: University of California Press.
Guttman, Samuel
1985 "The psychoanalytic point of view: basic concepts and deviant theories. A brief communication", *International Journal of Psychoanalysis* 66,167-170.
Habermas, Jürgen
1988 *On the logic of the social sciences.* (Translated by Shierry Weber Micholsen & Jerry A. Stark.) Cambridge MA: MIT Press.
Hartmann, Heinz
1964 *Understanding and explorations in essays on ego psychology.* New York: International Universities Press.
Kohut, Heinz
1984 *How does analysis cure?* Chicago IL: University of Chicago Press.
Kuhn, Thomas
1970 *The structure of scientific revolution.* (2nd edition.). Chicago IL: University of Chicago Press.

Lewis, C.J.
1952 "The given element in empirical knowledge", *Philosophical Review* 61, 168–175.
Lichtenberg, Joseph
1983 *Psychoanalysis and infant research.* Hillsdale NJ: The Analytic Press.
Peterfreund, Emanuel
1971 *Information, systems, and psychoanalysis: an evolutionary biological approach to psychoanalytic theory.* Psychological Issues VII nos. 1/2. New York: International Universities Press.
Piaget, Jean & Bärbel Inhelder
1969 *The psychology of the child.* New York: Basic Books.
Rorty, Richard
1989 *Contingency, irony and solidarity.* Cambridge: Cambridge University Press.
Rubovitz-Seitz, Philip
1986 "Clinical interpretation, hermeneutics, and the problem of validity", *Psychoanalysis and Contemporary Thought* 9, 3–42.
Schafer, Roy
1975 "Psychoanalysis without psychodynamics", *International Journal of Psychoanalysis* 56, 41–55.
Schimek, Jean
1975 "A critical re-examination of Freud's concept of unconscious mental representation", *International Review of Psychoanalysis* 2, 171–187.
Spence, Donald
1986 "When interpretation masquerades as explanation", *Journal of the American Psychoanalytic Association* 34, 13–22.
Stern, Daniel
1985 *The interpersonal world of the infant.* New York: Basic Books.
Stolorow, Robert & Bernard Brandchaft
1987 "Developmental failure and psychic conflict", *Psychoanalytic Psychology* 4, 241–253.
Stroud, B.
1974 *The significance of philosophical scepticism.* Oxford: Clarendon Press.
Warnke, Georgia
1987 *Gadamer. hermeneutics, tradition and reason.* Stanford CA: Stanford University Press.
Winnicott, Donald W.
1965 *The maturational processes and the facilitating environment.* New York: International Universities Press.

Semiosis and its "other": notes on the psychoanalytic unconscious

Barnaby B. Barratt

The rise of semiotic science during this century makes it seem possible for us to study every human event (by which I mean every event that exists for us, the human subjects studying the event) as a set of signs, a subsystem of the universe that is significant. The subatomic organization of quanta, the biochemical organization of neuroleptic effects, the psychological organization of an ego's defensive-adaptive functioning, the behavioral/material organization of an automobile manufacturing plant, the economic organization of trade in jute, and the international organization of global politics may all be considered as sign subsystems of various sorts. Such considerations immediately empower our analyses of the world, holding out the possibility of principles of organization inferable across different types or levels of significatory subsystems, promising to facilitate communication between researchers from different fields, and suggesting that all subsystems are part of the consistency of the grand totality of interconnected subsystems – that the knowable universe is one, and that we live and make our inquiries within the governance of an overarching system of semiotic law and order. For if signs are marks of identity/difference relations, then it seems unarguable that they always occur within an apparently preconstituted network of possibilities for such relations, and that these possibilities are governed by a general law and order of actual and potential relatedness, a totality of such actualities and potentialities. The intent of "science" is thus to articulate, by one means or another, the workings of this overarching system of law and order – to constitute, so to speak, a powerful significatory metacomment on the significatory workings of the universe in which we live.

Mainstream psychology and psychiatry have seen a shift in recent decades towards a wholly "cognitivist" program of investigation and model-building. Whereas it had been common to study affect, motivation, cognition, and behavior as if they were relatively distinct functions, nowadays all such matters are likely to be discussed in terms of their cognitive structuring, their regulation by schematic organizations, their informational processing properties, the modifiability of their implied neural networks, and so forth. It is now generally believed that such an approach has the capacity eventually to integrate the diversity of psychological events in a single explanatory paradigm. This shift to cognitivism emerged in the fifties, gained ground with the decline of behaviorist ideology, and triumphed conspicuously in this last decade. Although rarely discussed in this manner, in a certain sense this program follows from, and is a part of, the rise of semiotic science. For what are "schematic organizations" and the like if not a matter of signs and their systemic organization? In large measure, therefore, psychology and psychiatry have become part of this "semiotic revolution".

Psychoanalytic theorizing too has been influenced by the ascendance of the cognitivist program. Since the sixties, there have been several attempts to reinterpret psychoanalytic "models of the mind" in such terms (for example, the work of Colby, Erdelyi, Peterfreund and many others). Such ventures in "bridge-building" may be of considerable interest to us, although, as this paper will suggest indirectly, there are fundamental problems with the assumptions of such enterprises – just as there are problems with the supposition that all mental life can be treated as a matter of signs and their systemic organization, a supposition which will be the eventual focus of this paper.

Historically, it is interesting that, starting at the turn of the century and growing steadily to the present, semiotics and psychoanalysis develop more or less contemporaneously, and in parallel fashion. As is well known, psychoanalysis develops from Sigmund Freud's discovery of the *dynamic unconscious* – a dimensionality of mental life that is not captured by conscious reflection and yet influences every form and content which consciousness takes. Although psychoanalysis today may involve much besides this discovery, my assumption here is that the notion of the dynamic unconscious (which I shall later define and discuss) continues to be the discipline's distinguishing feature. Freud's discovery of the dynamic unconscious dates from approximately 1896, and is adumbrated in his great methodological works (e.g., 1898, 1899, 1900, 1901, 1904). More or less contemporaneously, semiotics develops from the major work of Charles Sanders Peirce. It is then augmented by the emergence of structural linguistics following Ferdinand de Saussure's influential Parisian lectures (1906-1911) as well as the subsequent rise of the so-called "structuralist movement" (Jakobson in Prague, Lévi-Strauss and others in Paris, Hjelmslev in Copenhagen, Bloomfield in the United States, and so on). And these developments in semiotics are later joined by the rise of cognitivism in psychology and psychiatry.

Taking them as merely parallel historical developments, one would be compelled to mention the recent "crosscurrents" between psychoanalysis and semiotics: for example, the appropriation of structural linguistics in Lacanian psychoanalysis, or the use of information processing models by which psychoanalysis might be assimilated to "cognitivism" (cf. Colby & Stoller 1988; Erdelyi 1985; Peterfreund 1971). However, I am less interested in this sort of intellectual history, the account of developments that seem to run in parallel, and more interested in the idea that psychoanalysis has been, from the very start, a semiotic discipline of a certain special sort (and I would argue this despite the fact that few psychoanalytic practitioners think of themselves in this manner, and even though many psychoanalysts have little familiarity with the discipline of semiotics as such).

Whatever the terminology involved, and whatever the self-understanding of its practitioners, psychoanalysis is a semiotic science because it is concerned with *signification* – with many and varied sorts of signs, with constructions and communications, with discourse, representationality, or "meanings" and their vicissitudes. In this paper, I shall present the argument that psychoanalysis is a semiotic discipline, but I shall also suggest how psychoanalysis contributes something unique and critical to the general study of semiotics. Concerned both with the semiosis of consciousness and with the semiosis of the discourse that pertains between the patient and the psychoanalyst, the critical uniqueness of psychoanalytic semiotics involves the way in which its method confronts the conditions and limits of our potential knowledge of signs, and of what signs are. In brief, I shall suggest that psychoanalytic method works through what is *other* than signification and its systemic organization, and that it thereby constitutes a critique of some of the major assumptions and methods of the general semiotic sciences (of structuralism, of cognitivism, and indeed of "modern science" itself).

To study signs in the manner of *modern science* (by which I mean "science" as defined within the analytico-referential "episteme", the episteme that has governed Western thinking from the Copernican-Galilean revolution to this century) is to proceed in one or both of two directions. On the one side, the sign subsystem can be studied as object, its functioning described translatively and its mode of organization inductively or deductively inferred. This is what we conventionally view as "science" (the science of microphysics, of biochemistry, of ego-psychology, and so on). On the other side, it can be studied as the condition by which such "objects" signify for us, the condition of the subject or consciousness that can study such events, and can itself be taken for reflexive and reflective interrogation. That is to say, there can be an inquiry as to how consciousness organizes the experience and understanding of signs, or, perhaps more precisely, how signs manifest themselves as consciousness – the way signs produce a subject that itself studies other signs. Such an inquiry is conventionally viewed as the province of philosophy (for example, the program of Kantian "analytic" epistemology, or the phenomenological investigation of the ego-subject that makes possible any experience or understanding). However, proceeding in either of these directions, analytico-referential science requires – and assumes – a subject that is unitary, the epistemological subject of the "scientific" consciousness, that can, by its apparent reiterativity, anchor the rationality of its observations and inferences, its discourse thereby claiming to apprehend the world in a logic or rhetoric of propositions that are noncontradictory or *identitarian.*

In this way, "modern science" has assumed the transparency of its articulations, their potential referentiality and rationality with respect to things that are held to exist external to their logical or rhetorical representation, the potential coincidence of language and logic, as well as the reiterative fixity, the unity, of the articulative subject of such representationalities – a "scientific" consciousness that can "know what it is talking about". As is well known, the doctrines of realism embedded in these epistemics, the supposition that language can designate existents outside of language itself (that words refer to "real" things and not just to other words, for example, or that representations actually "represent" a presence that is not itself a representation), have been a source of continuous philosophical debate for several centuries. However, the identitarianism of subject and representationality, the supposition that language accords with the consciousness of its enunciation (that the subject of reason and the semiotic mediating system, which the subject articulates and is articulated by, are united temporally and noncontradictorily at the moment of enunciation, for example, or that "I" can know what "I mean" when I articulate a meaning) is a fundament of these epistemics that went unchallenged from Descartes' meditations on its significance until the turn of this century. Freud's revolutionary impetus is precisely a challenge to this Cartesian ground on which all certainty can supposedly be constructed – at least according to Descartes and the "analytic" tradition of Cartesian-Kantian philosophy of science that follows him. In short, psychoanalytic method subverts the assumption that consciousness can ever "know what it is talking about", that the subject of semiosis, of representationality and meaning, can ever be coincident with the meanings it articulates, that the apparent identitarianism of consciousness (supposedly guaranteed by its operations of reflection) is ever a fixity, or reiterativity, by which analytico-referential knowledge might be secured.

Without being facetious it might be said that what is surely remarkable about signs is that they make themselves manifest to us – that signs appear to us as the consciousness of signs, seemingly always available either as if by some direct apprehension or by more indirect and complex modes of ratiocination, induction and deduction, analysis and synthesis. To express this differently, it could be said that if there are signs that are entirely unavailable to consciousness as signs, inherently unknowable, then they are not of any significance: at least, so we readily assume (and in what sense this assumption should be granted is under debate, by implication, at the end of this paper). Marx seems to have articulated something similar in his 1844 manuscripts: consciousness may always be of things represented, but "things" are also to be comprehended as consciousness made concrete (cf. Kolakowski 1968). In this century, with the so-called "linguistic turn" in philosophy (cf. Rorty 1967), as well as the development of semiotic sciences, increasingly the tendency is to equate existence with semiosis, or at least to equate what is accessible about existence with the law and order of semiosis. Supposedly, the world of "things", *being*, exists for us only as a totality of signification – the universe of signs is "all that is" or (to recall Peirce) "for us that is absolutely all there is in it." However, we might venture also that "nature," the world of "all that is", for us is constituted only out of our consciousness of it. The conditions and limits of semiotic science are – obviously – entirely bound to the conditions and limits of consciousness as the manifestation of semiosis. While there has been a general assumption in modern science (especially with the linguistic turn and with the development of semiotics) that signification and its consciousness are identitarian, and that meaning and the enunciation of meaning are temporally united as a foundational identicality, psychoanalysis subverts this metaphysics of idenitarianism.

Thus, in discussing semiosis (whether of quanta, of neuroleptic effects, of ego functioning, or whatever), one eventually arrives at discussion of the consciousness of semiosis, and the constraints on our ability to "know" signs or to "know" much about the conditions and limits of our knowledge. But precisely at the juncture of this discussion – of our consciousness of signification and of the way in which signification constitutes our consciousness – psychoanalysis intervenes dramatically on our notion of science itself, radically challenging our basic assumptions about matters of signification, reality, consciousness, temporality and truth. In this context then, I shall now turn to psychoanalysis itself. After intimating something of the character of the "discovery" of the dynamic unconscious, I shall present some interpretations of this discovery that are variously problematic. This section of the paper will focus principally on a *topographic interpretation* and then deal more briefly with interpretations offered by Lacan and by Kristeva. In the last section of this paper, I shall sketch a different line of interpretation, indicating what I take to be the radical significance of Freud's discovery (a discovery which, as we shall see, is actually never "discovered") and I shall sketchily show some of its implications for our notions of semiosis and semiotic inquiry.

1. "Discovering" the incomprehensible in our midst

The beginning of psychoanalysis as a science involves a method in which consciousness is encouraged to enunciate itself more or less "freely". Under these conditions of "free-associative" process – a relaxation of the restraints of propriety and of "making good sense", as well as an attempt to speak publicly all that "comes to mind" privately – it is readily found that the "I" of consciousness is incessantly mobile and that it never quite knows "what it is talking about". Here I will offer a vignette from my own practice, one that is – from the standpoint of a psychoanalytic practitioner – quite commonplace. I have discussed it twice elsewhere in somewhat different contexts (Barratt 1985, 1990). The vignette is, of course, edited and greatly simplified in order to be presentable and discussable here, but such modifications should not affect the way such an illustration bears on the gist of my argument.

What I shall describe took place during the first few minutes of a Monday session towards the end of this man's first year of psychoanalytic treatment. Here I should mention that, on the previous Friday, I had drawn the patient's attention to his repeated forgetting of the payment for the preceding month's treatment, and I suggested (gently, so I felt) that, in these actions (forgetting that payment was due, forgetting to write the check, writing the check and then failing to deliver it, and so forth), he might be expressing some hostility towards me and our work together. To this comment, the patient responded, as he often did to such interventions, with a sort of joking denial.

At the beginning of the next session, the patient reported that he had been anxious or "edgy" since his Friday appointment, and did not know why. Moreover, he indicated that he had entirely forgotten the themes and topics of that session as well as the entire previous week of psychoanalytic work: he was puzzled by this. What then came to mind was an event over the weekend. His young son had been mad at him and eventually, deciding that he could not deal with it, the patient left to spend several hours in a local bar. I shall call this S(1) (S standing for 'surfacing', for 'story', for 'set of signs' or 'symbolizations', for 'a syntactic/semantic/pragmatic event' for 'succession of associations', or whatever). Following S(1), the patient suddenly found himself thinking of something he had not recalled in years; and it bewildered him that this should then "come to mind". He became tearful as he recalled the Rabbi who had tutored him for his Bar Mitzvah around the time of his father's illness. This Rabbi had been very close with the patient as a boy, and was a figure of considerable importance in his life at that time. However, some month's after the Bar Mitzvah, the patient had become angry at the Rabbi over some disappointment and the latter had abruptly dropped the relationship, never again talking with the patient. I shall call this S(2). What next sprang into the patient's mind was his previous night's dream, one that he had forgotten on waking and only recalled at that moment. In the dream, he reported, we were happily walking together in some pleasant countryside, being very friendly towards each other – in this dream, he and I were, so he informed me, like "bosom buddies". I shall call the recounting of this dream S(3).

Here is a very brief succession or set of associations that play out a scenario brought to the fore, I would believe, by my remark at the end of the previous session, when I said something thematically along the lines of: "You may be beginning to experience some angry feelings towards me." Now *retrodictively*, it is very easy to suggest that the patient must have heard this remark (consciously or "preconsciously") as if it were accompanied by a contingent proposition: "If/when I express anger towards my psychoanalyst, then he will reject me." But note here, both my emphasis on the retrodictive quality of this inference, and that we cannot know whether the patient was indeed momentarily conscious of such an extended meaning, just that he subsequently acts as if he were operating on the assumption of such a contingency. What we do know is that he brushes aside my comment, and that, according to his subsequent report, he forgot all that had taken place, becoming anxious throughout the weekend.

Let us now consider S(1), S(2) and S(3). They are preceded by the patient's questioning along the lines of: "Why have I been anxious since Friday's session?" The "answer" to this question both "arrives" and fails to "arrive" in the shifting from S(1) to S(3). S(1) might then be characterized as follows: "When (in the recent past) my son was angry at me, then I rejected him (leaving for the bar)." S(2) might plausibly be characterized as follows: "When (in the distant past) I was angry at the Rabbi, then he rejected me (and I am tearful yet do not know why)." S(3) might be summarized as follows: "Closely and happily, you and I are together (in recent dreamtime, in the wish, in the past, in the present, in the future, forever?)." Obviously my characterizations of these three "stories" are open to amendment and alteration; and equally obviously there is much more at issue in these associations than I am about to discuss (even with respect to this edited version of the patient's discourse I am going to omit discussion of the significance of the patient's mentioning bars, Bar Mitzvahs, the death of his father, the affective tone of the dream's countryside, and the connotations of "bosom buddiness"). However, what I hope is compelling in this illustration is the way in which free-associative process is a movement of thinking and speaking that, in each moment of its enunciations and transitions, both conceals and reveals, concomitantly and concurrently, something other than what it (as the conscious awareness of the moment) is talking about manifestly. Moreover, I would argue that this method of psychoanalytic discourse, the "work-play" of the process, merely serves to exhibit consciousness as such: that free-associative process is what consciousness is, the mobility of a contradictorious compositioning.

For example, drawing on the *retrodictive scenario* ("if/when I express anger towards my psychoanalyst, then he will reject me"), we might reach some of the following conclusions. S(1) expresses the anger/rejection contingency but otherwise disguises the retrodictive scenario by talking about an event cast in the recent past instead of the here and now, by talking about the son instead of the psychoanalyst, and by reversing the positions of agent and recipient in both the anger and the rejection phases of the story. S(2) again expresses the anger/rejection contingency and moves further towards the story of the retrodictive scenario by positioning the patient himself as the agent in the anger phase and the recipient in the rejection phase of the story (and perhaps also by the occurrence of an eruption of affect that is inexplicable to the patient). However, at the very same time, S(2) further disguises the retrodictive scenario by talking about an event cast in the far more distant past instead of the here and now, as well as by talking about a Rabbi with whom the patient says he has had no contact for many years instead of talking about the psychoanalyst or even the son (and perhaps also by the occurrence of an eruption of affect that is inexplicable to the patient). Then, the shifting from S(2) to S(3) dramatically moves to a story that is closer to my retrodictive scenario in that the patient and the psychoanalyst are the protagonists in the here and now of a dream report (which is an anomalous timeframe, referring ambiguously to a wished-for time, maybe also a feared-for time, a dreamtime present, a potential present, a future, and maybe even a figurative past). But of course, S(3) then also dramatically moves further away from my retrodictive scenario by abolishing the contingency of anger/rejection, erasing the positionalities of agent and recipient, and asserting the prevalence of a pleasant affective tone, of togetherness, friendliness, and bosom buddiness.

In these transitions from S(1) to S(3) there is the restlessness of a revealing-concealing movement in which each enunciation "stands for" manifestly "what it is talking about" (what the story purports to be about and takes itself to be about, what the consciousness of the subject that enunciates it knows it to be about, by means of this subject's reflective awareness). And yet each enunciation also expresses disguisedly an excess of meaningfulness, a remainder that contradicts its sense of itself, a trace or *différance*, the mark of something "otherwise" than that which "makes sense", a nonidenticality of meaningfulness that subverts the narratological unity or completion and closure of the story as such-subverting the governance of the syntactic/semantic/ pragmatic law and order that creates the story as such, as well as the epistemic privilege of the "I-ness" of its enunciation. The shifting from S(1) to S(2), for example, both reveals and conceals something other than either S(1) or S(2) make manifest, as does the shifting from S(2) to S(3). And S(2), the story of the Rabbi, expresses disguisedly something other than that which it purports to be about and takes itself to be about, yet is not consciously or deliberatively selected or created as allegory or trope. The subject that enunciates the saga of the Rabbi – the "I-ness" of consciousness that can reiteratively produce and reproduce the "I is I" of consciousness – does not know what it also expresses disguisedly, and even if this subject believes that it knows why it is thinking and speaking that which it thinks and speaks, the adequacy of this "why" is immediately contradicted by the persistence and insistence with which the Rabbi story issues into the remembrance of the dream.

To be more precise, taken as a moment of the subject's discourse, the construction and communication of the Rabbi story presents multiple, manifest meanings.

S(2) presents meanings that are *factual* (the patient knows that he thinks these events happened), *interpersonal* (the patient knows he expects some sort of response from the psychoanalyst, his audience, to the telling of the story; he expects his addressee to "get the point"), *thematic* (the patient knows that he believes the story to have a message, that there is a point to the story), and so forth. An entire network of rules determines these multiple types or levels of semiotic meaningfulness. These rules are what I am calling the totality of *semiotic law and order*, rules that may variously be defined or described as syntactic/semantic/pragmatic, informational or lexical, logical and rhetorical rules that "make sense" of events for us (makes an "event" as such), giving our sense of the world as meaningful – our sense of our own thinking as referentially correspondent and rationally coherent. And yet, as with any manifestation of consciousness, S(2) does not just make sense. In the midst of its comprehensible enunciation lies the incomprehensible. It is incongruous "within" (the patient becomes tearful and does not know why), and inconsistent "without" (the patient does not know why the saga comes to mind as it does, why it should issue from the son story nor why it should issue into the remembrance of the dream). In this way, the mobility of the subject, the movement from S(1) to S(2) to S(3) undermines the logical and rhetorical structuration of chronology/narratology and the unicity of representational temporality – the apparent reiterativity of signification. The mobility of this "sequence" subverts the privileging of manifest meaningfulness in all of its multiple types or levels (factual, interpersonal, thematic, and so on). It subverts the totalizing of the semiotic law and order by which the subject can appear to make sense. These subversions intimate the working-playing of the so-called "dynamic unconscious" – a working-playing which free-associative process best exhibits.

In sum, the disruptures of making sense intimate something other than the law and order that governs the structuration of making sense. This is the key to Freud's discovery. Like all enunciations of consciousness, each S, as a moment of the patient's discourse, conveys or is conveyed by the dynamic unconscious. Its enunciation or manifestation is, disguisedly expressed, a "return of the repressed" (cf. Barratt 1984). Here, something is "in" the subject's thinking and speaking yet not "of" the semiotics of the subject's constructions and communications. Something "other" reveals-conceals itself through (and yet against) the jurisdictions and determinations of semiotic law and order, the reiterative temporality of the present's presencing as signification.

2. Interpreting the "dynamic unconscious"

If the above illustrates the process of free-associative work-play that Freud (1931: 403) called "the methodological key" to psychoanalysis, what does it suggest to us about the semiotics of consciousness? And how are we to grasp the so-called "discovery of the dynamic unconscious"? Here I will survey some of the major lines of response to these questions, ways of comprehending Freud's discovery, that have in various forms preoccupied psychoanalytic theorizing since the turn of the century. I am not suggesting that the survey is complete, that these modes of comprehension have been the only available ways of theorizing Freud's dynamic unconscious, or that they are necessarily incompatible with each other. But I do hold that such a survey, even if oversimplified, will prove helpful polemically and pedagogically, and will provide a backdrop for my introduction of a different way of thinking – my discussion of consciousness and its subject, which has, I believe, some radical implications for our thinking about the question of science, the metaphysics of time, and the general study of semiosis.

The first way of theorizing the dynamic unconscious I will call the *topographic*. It is Freud's first response to the study of free-associative process, ably documented in several essays (e.g., 1912, 1915a, 1915b, 1933), and discussed by many subsequent commentators of which Rapaport (1960) is one of the more adept. Although there is a widespread opinion (particularly among American psychoanalysts) that the subsequent development of the structural-functional model of the mind (the ego's formation of conscious representations as "compromises" with the demands of the id, the superego, and reality) came to supercede topographic theorizing, the latter is embedded in the structural-functional model in such a way that my remarks here will also pertain in large measure to contemporary theorizing in the American tradition of ego-psychology (the influential tradition of Anna Freud, Hartmann, Rapaport, Arlow, Brenner, and their followers).

The topographic interpretation depicts the dynamic unconscious as if it were spatial, a region of the mind in which there are stored representations (thoughts, feelings, wishes) that have been at some previous time "repressed", and which cannot be deliberatively accessed by the subject of consciousness. It is presumed that such representations were once consciously enunciated and were subsequently repressed into this unconscious. Once "in" the repressed unconscious, the organization of their storage is anomalous: most saliently, common arrangements of logic, rhetoric, and the temporal rules of chronology do not pertain. Yet more importantly, such representations neither deteriorate nor remain ineffectual. Rather, it must be supposed that they not only persist unmodified since their repression, but also insist by attempting to influence the form and content of those representations that are enunciated by the subject of consciousness (and this persistence and insistence gives consciousness its recondite character as the "return of the repressed", manifest meanings being the condensed and displaced expression of an allegedly "latent" core of repressed thoughts, feelings and wishes).

Thus, with my illustration, the topographic interpretation would suggest that there exists "in the patient's unconscious" a representation, a proposition the form and content of which might be something like my retrodictive scenario ("if/when I express anger towards my psychoanalyst, then he will reject me"). Let us call this proposition S(u). The topographic interpretation is thus that the existence of S(u) in the unconscious determines the sequential production and reproduction in consciousness of S(1), S(2) and S(3). Or, under a different description, S(1), S(2) and S(3) are each determined, in their form and content, as translations by means of condensation and displacement (metaphoric and metonymic transformations) of some "latent" organizing representation, namely S(u). Moreover, at the time in which S(1), S(2) and S(3) are enunciated by the subject of consciousness, this subject cannot articulate the presencing (the persistence and insistence) of S(u) upon its own constructions and communications. Indeed, the premise is that, if S(u) were told to the patient and eventually integrated into the successive enunciations of his consciousness, then it would lose its determinate influence on the organization of representational production and reproduction in consciousness: "the unconscious" would have been brought to consciousness, perhaps.

There is much in favor of the topographic interpretation. For example, it is clinically heuristic, for it is difficult for a beginning psychoanalyst (or a beginning patient) to tolerate free-associative process, and consequently, the psychoanalyst is liable either to lapse into something antipsychoanalytic and anticurative (such as wanting the patient to "make good sense") or to anchor the process by formulating some interim organizing principles by which the psychoanalyst can at least privately believe that "good sense" can be made of the patient's capricious and fluctuating discourse even while the patient does not recognize it. The topographic formulation of a retrodictive scenario believed to be S(u) by the psychoanalyst provides such an anchor (although I would argue that such formulations, even when held only privately, are also subtly antipsychoanalytic and anticurative). Alongside this heuristic aspect of the topographic interpretation (and also in its favor) is that the retrodictive scenario, when specified, can be very compelling: as with my illustration, we may, too readily, come to believe that S(u) is "what the patient really means" when he says S(1), S(2) and S(3). Moreover, the patient may sooner or later arrive at the enunciation of the retrodictive scenario himself, or he may be told it by the psychoanalyst and then adopt it, coming to believe himself that this was "really" why he said what he said. And such apparent "vindications" of the retrodictive scenario too easily (but by an erroneous path of reasoning) lead us to believe that S(u) must therefore have been "in" the patient's unconscious when he said what he said, as a hidden representation that animated the transitions (now to be comprehended not as disruptures but as transformations within some overarching scheme) between those representations which were manifested by conscious enunciation. Of course, there is here (and it is an issue around which Grünbaum has recently created such a controversy in the psychoanalytic literature) a sort of perverted *post hoc, ergo propter hoc* argument: namely, if S(u) comes after S(1), S(2) and S(3) and renders them into a convincingly consistent sequence, then it must have been there existent "unconsciously" at the time of the enunciation of S(1), S(2) and S(3) as the reason for their "coming to mind" and as their "latent" organizing principle or determinant (their "cause" perhaps).

Here lies the persuasiveness of the retrodictive scenario, disposing us towards a belief in the existence of S(u) in a topographic unconscious. Even though it is retrodictive, as I emphasized earlier, and founded on a kind of back-to-front reasoning, the topographic interpretation can be convincing precisely because it appears to restore (fallaciously, ideologically) the shifting of S(1) to S(3) to the law and order of logical and rhetorical governance. For example, it recasts disruptive transitions as rule-bound transformations, shiftings as sequences, and so on. It recasts the succession of apparently meaningless transitions (recondite to the "I" of their enunciation) into a set of apparently meaningful transformations. And it does so by specifying a wider frame within which everything still appears to make sense – since we want to believe that everything ultimately will make sense, we too readily agree that, if the text of S(2), for example, is not fully comprehensible, then it must become so by contextualizing it expansively until a narratological enclosure of the frame, a full version that makes sense, appears to be attained. But aside from the problem of a kind of back-to-front reasoning that I just mentioned, two points about the epistemology of this topographic interpretation should be noticed.

First, with the imperative to restore the semiotic law and order of "making sense", the care for the subject of consciousness, the concern with what the "I" is and what it can know, has actually been abandoned. We, the capital purveyors of "science", now claim to make sense of the patient's enunciations by "translating" or recontextualizing them, formulating a public (objective, intersubjective, hermeneutically consensual) version of the patient's words in which their disruptures and discontinuities have now been rendered nugatory or expunged; but "we" can only do so retrodictively, by passing over the contradictoriness of the moment itself, which is a passing over of the subject itself, the being of the subject as a contradictorious locus of mobility that is an enunciatory movement which never knows fully "what it is talking about". This "passing over" is an imposing, impositioning or imprisoning of the subject by the (re)structuration of normative discourse, the hegemony of the unicity of representational time (to be discussed later). The justification for such a treatment of the subject reverts (amongst other aspects) to an ideology of adaptation: the subject must be positioned and repositioned more adaptively within the communal standards of making sense (even by perpetuation and intensification of this subject's alienation). This therapeutic goal then obliterates our caring for the free-associative subject, the subject as it "is", a contradictory locus of transmutation and truthfulness.

Second, it must be noted how the topographic interpretation retains its coherence (and its semblance of corresponding to something existent "in" the unconscious yet outside of the conscious subject's realm of the retrievable or recognizable) by an appeal to the notion that everything ultimately must make sense semiotically, that everything meaningful must be meaningful in terms of the law and order of representationality. This is an appeal to a telos, the reflected totality of signification as "all that is" significant, and it requires, as I shall later suggest, metaphysical assumptions about the unicity of time, time as the unitary time of representational reiterativity. But such assumptions are called into question by psychoanalytic method itself.

The very persuasiveness of the topographic interpretation, its availability to the commonsense of making sense, might itself be a reason to examine it with suspicion. That it is persuasive should not convince us that it is epistemologically sound (as I have just suggested), nor that mental life actually operates in the manner it specifies. In relation to the latter, there are several problems with the model of the mind derived from the topographic interpretation. I will mention some of these. Each has been discussed in the psychoanalytic literature and although I cannot review these discussions in the brevity of this paper, I will indicate why I do not find the various "defenses" of the topographic interpretation adequate.

The foremost problem is perhaps the one first encountered by Freud himself: if representations (now depicted as substantial) are shunted around the mind (now depicted as spatial), from its surface to its hypothetical "depth" and back, then there has to be an account of the agency or "mechanism" of the shunting (the repressing, the returning of the repressed, and so forth). As is well known, Freud resolved this by speculations about *energy*, leading to further problems as to the agency of the energy. For example, how would a formless, contentless energy "know" which representations (representations having form and content) to pour itself into, which to push into the area of the unconscious, and which to allow to consciousness? In terms of conventional epistemology, the attempted solution to this has been to jettison the energy idea and formulate an entirely cognitivist model in which there are only representations (thoughts, feelings, wishes) and their transformations. The topography of conscious/unconscious regions is then partly salvaged in terms of the specification of two orders of representational organization – but this itself leads to further difficulties, as I will indicate.

Another problem stems from the depiction of the topographic unconscious as containing representations that are meaningful more or less in the manner that conscious representations are meaningful. For example, S(u) is held to have the form and content of a proposition. The issue then is that, when "in" the unconscious, these propositions both persist unmodified and yet are no longer organized according to the common rules of logic, rhetoric and chronological time (the regimented, unitary, linear and equable time of semiotic reiterativity). This leads to difficulties in depicting the relation between the conscious organization and the unconscious – the transformations involved in the action of repressing these propositions and in the action of their returning. For example, how does a representation that is rule-bound get transformed into one that is not, yet retain its potential for a meaningfulness that can influence the domain of rule-bound representationality? Or, to be yet more simplistic, how would an illogical, catachrestic and quasi-timeless representation "know" to which conscious (logical, rhetorical, chronological) representation to attach itself, to (dis)organize or determine? In terms of conventional epistemology, one effort at a solution to this has been to delineate two distinct (but interrelated) modes of thinking, namely *primary* and *secondary process*. This attempt, begun by Freud, has been further developed by several talented commentators. It does not, however, resolve the epistemological difficulties, nor does it actually rescue the topographical model of the mind – since either one specifies two regions each of which deploys one of the two processes exclusively, in which case the above difficulties pertain; or one argues that the two processes are always inmixed, in which case the power of the topographic model disappears with other difficulties arising in its stead. Another effort at a solution has been to suggest that all representationality is always metaphoric and metonymic, which might relieve S(u) of its privileged status as an organizing principle and determinant of S(1), S (2) and S(3). This is a quite successful line of argument – congenial to a "cognitivist psychoanalysis" – but one that effectively erases the main claims of the topographic interpretation, as well as raising further questions about the status of the subject, the "I" that is unknowingly carried along this chain of metaphors and metonyms, articulating the pathways of these successive condensations and displacements.

The ideas of change implied by the topographic interpretation are also problematic: the premise that enunciation of S(u) by the conscious subject will reduce the power of the unconscious over the ongoing formation of representations. There are two approaches to this. On the one side, it could be argued that S(u) is, by its conscious articulation, transferred from having been "in" the unconscious to being "in" the repertoire of conscious representations (now retrievable and recognizable by the "I" of consciousness); that is, the representation no longer exists in the unconscious because it has been made conscious (extricated from the unconscious, so to speak). In this argument, it seems to follow that the topographic unconscious, since it presumably contains a finite store of S(u) representations, could be "drained" out of existence (and Freud indeed suggested this). But many clinical reasons make this account implausible. On the other side, it could be argued that S(u) cannot be taken out of the topographic unconscious, but that it loses its influence on consciousness when it also becomes represented, or at least given a more or less equivalent representation, in the repertoire of conscious articulation (giving rise to a sort of "double registration" as Freud suggested at least once). However, in this argument, it is unclear why the articulation of a conscious representation along the lines of S(u) (an "in-sight" into the unconscious, so to speak) should cause the unconscious S(u) to cease insisting itself on the conscious subject, especially since the multiple articulation of conscious representations which are supposedly condensations and displacements of S(u) fails to have such a taming effect on the "stuff" of the unconscious. All this may sound absurdly anthropomorphic (a mythography of an unconscious realm with an unconscious subject of its disordered representationality facing adversatively a conscious realm with a conscious subject of its ordered representationality), but it is precisely into such anthropomorphism that the topographic interpretation inevitably embroils us.

The topographic interpretation of the dynamic unconscious fails. But, contrary to some opinions, this does not imply that there is no such discovery. This interpretation fails even while it is clinically heuristic and superficially persuasive (and I would argue similarly that the structural-functional model is clinically heuristic but scientifically and philosophically untenable). There has been, from the start, an ideological subterfuge in the formulation of the topographic unconscious, and this subterfuge has two aspects. First, the topographic interpretation is a depiction of life in which everything remains within the bounds of semiotic law and order, everything appears ultimately comprehensible – except the subject itself that must be overlooked. This depiction fails utterly to account for the subject of discourse, to account for the contradictoriness of the subject's enunciations, the "I" that breaks open the unity of representational time at the very moment of the articulation of the "I-now-is". Or, under another description, the topographic model fails to account for the way in which the totality of semiotic law and order could produce and reproduce a subject that contradicts itself at the very moment of its enunciation. Second, the topographic interpretation, by rendering the unconscious as a region existing apart from (but impacting upon) the domain of consciousness, ideologically preserves the potential for consciousness to operate, at least on occasions, without the distorting intrusions of unconscious thoughts, feelings or wishes. This rescues, so it might seem, the ideology of a rational and unified subject that can on some occasions (such as when the community agrees that this is so) know fully "what it is talking about". The "scientific consciousness" required by the modern episteme thereby appears to be defended, the dichotomy of subject/object necessary to all the epistemologies of modern "science" is thereby reinstated – for if the realm of the unconscious is "outside" the domain of consciousness, then it is not always "inside", and thus consciousness may proceed confident of its capacity eventually to represent in full, to dominate, conquer and possess that which is "without". However, against this "defense" of the modern episteme, it must be said that the topographic interpretation is not viable, and the seriousness of the challenge that psychoanalysis makes to the prevailing assumptions about the subject, consciousness and the possibilities of knowing, has yet to be realized.

The second way of theorizing the dynamic unconscious I will call the *Lacanian*. I do not mean that what follows stands as a sufficient account of the intricacies of Lacanian psychoanalysis, but rather that it is drawn from Lacan's writings and is the aspect of my reading of Lacan that seems pertinent to this paper (cf. Lacan 1964, 1977, 1988a, 1988b). Lacan insists that the subject of consciousness cannot be considered apart from its enunciations, the "I-ness" of S(1), S(2) and S(3), but that this subject is forever decentered from itself because it is structured – its utterances are produced and reproduced – from "elsewhere", that is, from the *symbolic order* as the capitalized *Other* which is the unconscious. The *sine qua non* of the Lacanian interpretation of Freud's discovery is thus the structuralist idea of the symbolic order now redescribed as Other. He supposes that the Other operates according to the rules of a completed and closed system – a totality by which all the possibilities for pathways of semiotic meaning, for chains of metaphor and metonym, are established, in the sense that there are immutable rules for the selection, combination and permutation of signs. The Other is thus the law and order of semiosis, and this totality is assumed to be synchronic, universal, closed, and (at least as far as the subject of reflective consciousness is concerned) "always already given".

Since this structuration of signs determines all possibilities of thinking and speaking, the "I" of enunciation and exchange has no authorial prerogative; it is merely a particular signifier – although perhaps an exemplary one – that "glides" over the totality of the Other. According to Lacan, this Other is Freud's unconscious over which the subject's enunciation of S(1), S(2), S(3) and so forth glides. It is a transindividual realm of discourse, a geometric or morphological space, the rules of which might be algebraically definable (hence Lacan's interest in unusual topological geometries and the like). Most importantly, this Other is "neither being, nor non-being, but the unrealized" (1964: 30), having itself nothing other than itself, its totality bounded only by death. Given this, it is as if this unconscious Other is continually trying to realize itself by generating an other for itself in the being of the "I" of consciousness – the subject whose words it produces and reproduces. However, attempting this realization across the gap of death, the "lack of being" of the Other, it is forever unsuccessful: the subject it creates is always and forever faulted. Moreover, the subject itself can never restore the "lost" continuity of its consciousness precisely because its words are never its own – being produced and reproduced from the "elsewhere" that is the law and order of the Other.

Given this Lacanian metaphysics, the Other (the unconsciousness of semiotic law and order as the unrealized totality of meaningfulness) and the subject (the "I" of consciousness or enunciation) are depicted in an endlessly circular, and yet peculiarly lopsided relation: the being of the "I-ness" of consciousness depends for its manifestation on what is produced and reproduced from the place of the Other, yet the latter can only generate the thinking/speaking subject as the signifier of its own absence or lack of being. This rift between the Other and its "I" is insurpassable. I shall not here enter into a debate with the Lacanian metaphysics in any detail, but shall merely raise some critical questions about Lacanian theorizing as an interpretation of the dynamic unconscious (although it will be seen that such questions always relate back to the metaphysical issues).

The foremost problem with Lacanian psychoanalysis – one on which there is a large literature, and to which I shall therefore give short shrift here – lies with Lacan's specific characterization of the Other as an immutably closed totality, as phallocentric and as logocentric. I have discussed the (phallo)logocentricity of this ontotheological design elsewhere, along with Lacan's commitment to an antidialectical notion of totality (Barratt 1984, forthcoming). Here I will merely point to the paradox by which Lacan insists that the knowledge of consciousness (the reflectivity of the "I") is always illusory (the "I" being a gliding signifier that does not constitute its own words), and yet he implies that a right-minded community of "men" might, by means of a calculus, come to know "what the Other is about". By this paradox, Lacan attempts both to dismiss the subject of enunciation as a pretentious trifle (the phantasmagory of Cartesian epistemology) and yet to preserve the propriety and privilege of a revamped, (phallo)logocentric "scientific consciousness".

A further problem arises concerning the transindividual character of the Other which implies, in a certain sense, that neither the unconscious nor the manifestations of consciousness have what might be called a "personal" significance. In a certain sense, both the notion of the repressed and, more crucially, the notion of consciousness as being a disguised expression of something other than that which it knows, a returning of the repressed, have disappeared from consideration. For example, it will be readily noticed that S(u) has no place in the Lacanian design (less noticeable, and yet more critical, is the way the notion of the moment of the conscious "I-now-is" as inherently contradictorious also has no place in this design). For Lacan, the unconscious Other is the law and order that produces and reproduces the signs that the "I" thinks or speaks. There are no signs in the unconscious itself, for the Other lacks being. And therefore the retrodictive scenario has no special priority, as just another metaphor/metonym in the endless chaining of signification (generated by the Other and uttered by the "I"). The "I" can never know "what it is talking about" because it never generates its own words, and the "knowledge" it claims by means of its reflectivity is illusory (*parole vide*, except for certain nodes which Lacan calls "anchoring points"). So, in a certain sense, not only does S(u) disappear and the retrodictive scenario become of no special interest, but also the character of S(1), S(2) and S(3) is actually of no special significance either – there is nothing to be gained, for example, by examining them objectively or subjectively. This gives the Lacanian "clinic" (as the Lacanians call their practice of treatment) its unusual features. The patient's stories are not of intrinsic interest, for there are no "insights" into the unconscious to be gained and no new stories concerning the patient to be created – such acquisitions of apparent knowledge stem from the *méconnaissance* of the "I" or ego and are condemned as merely a theater of the *imaginary register*. Rather, the program of the "clinic" is to bring about a certain awareness on the part of the subject – not the confident but spurious awareness of reflectively founded knowledge on the part of the epistemological ego – but an awareness of the "imaginary" character of what the "I" takes to be its own, an awareness of its own meaningfulness as actually being determined from "elsewhere".

But here Lacan seems to equivocate, for while he does insist that there is never anything the "I" can do to know (let alone to regulate or control) why it thinks and speaks what it thinks and speaks, he nonetheless holds out the idea that there are "anchoring points", occasional moments of identicality between the Other and the "I" at which the latter happens to enunciate "full" speech: in Schneiderman's (1989) phrasing, "I" can have the experience or understanding of "saying the right thing, at the right time, at the right place" even if only on rare occasions. But how could this be? Within the terms of Lacanian theorizing, it seems impossible to specify how "I" (the Lacanian patient or the Lacanian psychoanalyst) would ever know the occasions on which the "I" is supposedly enunciating full speech. How could the "I" discriminate full speech from *parole vide*? Or, if such a discrimination could indeed be made, would not the main edifice of theorizing about the relation between the Other and the "I" – which Lacan sets up so assiduously – collapse? There is a parallel problem here. If the "I" is without power, without the "authority" ever to create its own meaningfulness, and if the structuring of signification is entirely determined by the Other, then it is unclear, at least to me, how Lacanian theorizing accounts for the disruptures, the "lost" continuities, and the inconsistencies of the subject's discourse. To express this differently, the relations between what Lacan calls the "symbolic order" and the "imaginary register" are not sufficiently explicated. If the "I" has being but no capacity to produce or reproduce meaning, and this capacity belongs to the totalized law and order of the Other, why is discourse manifested in such medleys of contradiction?

The major terms in the Lacanian ontotheology are – in my phrasing – semiosis as a totality of meaning, being as the subject, and death. While this gives us an interesting account of the boundedness of signification by absence or lack of being, it seems that it is an effort to bypass the notion of contradictoriness in the ideological interests of keeping established the mandate of modern "science" – the honorific status of a "scientific consciousness" by which "men" can know the universe that is already assumed by them to be inexorably (phallo)logocentric in its structuration. Lacanian theorizing follows Heideggerian hermeneutic ontology in holding out the notion of *alétheia* as the union of veiling/unveiling which, as Derrida (1972c) has argued, suggests the stillness of a "truth" achievable through the potential presencing of being in the presentness of thinking and speaking. This notion is problematic, because it expunges what I take to be the radicalism of Freud's free-associative discovery, namely the contradictoriness of the locus of the "I" at every moment of its enunciation, and also because it serves ideologically to cast life within the unicity of the time of representationality (the Other as totality implying the enclosure of temporality as a unity). And, as I shall suggest, the metaphysics of a unitary time (the time of semiotic reiterativity and the hegemony of the notion of the presentness of the present as presencing) is precisely what the discovery of the dynamic unconscious would seem to break open.

The third way of theorizing the dynamic unconscious I will call the *Kristevan*. I believe Kristeva herself, as a practicing psychoanalyst, would see this interpretation of the unconscious as a modification of Lacanian theorizing. We might even aptly characterize it as a feminist amendment to the Lacanian design (except that Kristeva is suspicious of the label "feminist"). In her major writings, Kristeva (1969, 1974, 1977, 1980) discusses the *chora*, described by Plato as "an invisible and formless being which receives all things and in some mysterious way partakes of the intelligible, and is most incomprehensible" (*Timaeus* [1959:51]). For Kristeva (1974), the *chora* is equivalent to (or at least a major dimensionality of) the dynamic unconscious, which is "the mother and receptacle of all things". It is the (m)Other as a "nonexpressive totality formed by the drives and their stases in a motility that is as full of movement as it is regulated", but despite this "nonexpressiveness" the *chora* is also full of "extremely provisional articulations". In her view of signification, Kristeva thus makes a provocative distinction. On the one "side", there is the representationality of the symbolic order which produces and reproduces the subject as signifier, and which consists of thetic propositions, judgements, positionalities and the like, organized according to the "law of the father" – and giving us our sense of the intelligibility of the universe. On the other "side" (but perhaps always in-mixed), there are the "articulations" of the *chora*

(Kristeva calls this *le sémiotique* which I shall avoid here since it would only add terminological confusions to this paper). The latter are both "energy charges" and "psychical marks". She claims that such articulations are not signs in the proper sense, but the intimations of a mode of being – a bodily mode – that is, in a certain sense, "prior" to the dichotomies of subject/object, inside/outside or "me/not-me". However, these intimations somehow intervene inexhaustibly upon the productions and reproductions of the symbolic order resulting in the "radical heterogeneity" of the manifestations of discourse – as a "negativity" of "charges and stases" expressing itself within the domain of "making sense".

In this paper, I will not document further Kristeva's speculations about these "charges and stases" – her arguments that they are articulated by condensations and displacements, organized around the psychosexuality of the body, characterized by paths of sadism, the "death drive", or melancholy, and that they comprise a "heterogenous object" excluded or foreclosed by logical or rhetorical law and order, but nonetheless persistent and insistent upon the productions of this law and order. I will also not deal here with the influence on Kristeva's speculations of Klein's (1921-1963) discussions of pre-Oedipality, Deleuze and Guattari's (1972, 1980) ideas about the "destructuring and a-signifying machine of the unconscious", or Merleau-Ponty's (1964) notion of "chiasmic flesh". Rather I will simply appreciate the Kristevan interpretation for what it achieves, while raising some critical questions about its shortcomings.

The remarkable quality of the Kristevan interpretation of the dynamic unconscious is that it improves on both topographic and orthodox Lacanian interpretations. For example, it stands as an attempted remedy for the (phallo)logocentric assumptions on which Lacan develops his notion of the Other, and of Lacan's totalization of this Other in terms of the law and order of representationality – of "language" in the sense of natural languages. Against any totalization of the "law of the father", Kristeva advances her notion of the *chora* as (m)Other. As a remedy for the topographic interpretation, for example, Kristeva makes it clear that all meaningfulness is not a matter of representationality. Rather, she offers an account of the semiosis of the unconscious as of a different ordering from the intelligibility of the representational (but an ordering nevertheless). Thus, although the "charges and stases" emanating from the *chora* are excluded and foreclosed by the logical and rhetorical structuration of thinking or speaking, and even though they nonetheless somehow intervene on this structuration, she does not allow that they can be (re)appropriated by representational articulation – their meaningfulness is not translatable into the meaningfulness of representationality, they cannot be knowable as such, and thus are not available for territorialization by the subject of the symbolic order.

This brings us to the critical questions about the Kristevan interpretation. The foremost problem concerns her depiction of the *chora* in spatial or morphological terms. The notion of the unconscious as the being that is the "receptacle" containing the discourse of representationality – indeed, anterior to this discourse, in some speculative sense, and therefore outside of or autonomous from it – raises two major issues. The first concerns the significance of the meaningfulness emanating from the *chora* in relation to the subject's logical and rhetorical discourse, and the second concerns more general questions concerning the relation between the *chora* and the symbolic order of the subject. Difficulties can be anticipated here, since Plato had already suggested that this "receptacle" both partakes of – or participates in – all that is intelligible, yet remains mysterious and incomprehensible to the standards of intelligibility. Speculatively, Kristeva wants to present the unconscious *chora* as a place both anterior to and yet required for the emergence of symbolic thinking and speaking: a "presignificatory space" that nevertheless signifies, nonrepresentationally, by its interventions upon – and its negativity, its destructuring of – the structurations of logical and rhetorical meaningfulness.

Clearly, there are paradoxes here. For example, according to Kristeva, the "articulations" of the *chora* are not signs, neither unities nor identicalities, and do not privilege presence over absence in the identitarian manner of signs. Since the *chora* is neither a unity nor an identity (nor is it the deity, although Kristeva comes strikingly close to such a theology), its interventions upon the significations of the symbolic order, the domain of the "I", give the latter a "radical heterogeneity" it would presumably not have if it were purely governed by the logical or rhetorical law and order. However, Kristeva also wants to claim that the articulations of the *chora* are a modality of regulation *(réglementation)*, necessary to the homogeneity of the symbolic order (although she continues to try to avoid rendering the notion of the *chora* into an essentialism, an ontological essence, like a substratum, that mutely makes possible the maneuverings of representationality). Indeed, the articulations of the *chora* supposedly "facilitate" the symbolic order (albeit negatively via processes of schism, break and rupture), providing it with a receptacle whose charges and stases comprise a "structuring disposition". Here then is a paradox: the *chora* as receptacle, as disruptive negativity, and yet as necessary regulation.

Such paradoxes might not be troublesome were Kristeva able to discuss further how the "marks" of the *chora* intervene upon the domain of representationality (here, there are parallels with the problematic theorizing of primary and secondary process, mentioned above). However, where are "repression" and the "return of the repressed" in this interpretation? If repression is depicted here, it is as a destructuring: representations are not pushed into, or dragged down into, the space of the unconscious, as the topographic interpretation supposes, but they might be "destructured," their representationality erased and thus relegated to being the marks of the *chora*. However, such a repressed cannot be held to "return" to the discourse of consciousness in any sense that might be meaningful to its representationality: the subject of consciousness can only find meaningless the radical heterogeneity that intrudes on the homogeneity of its productions and reproductions. And yet Kristeva continues to write of the "transformation" from the "drives" of the *chora* to the "signifier" of the symbolic order, and "transformation" can only here imply their coincidence within the unicity of temporality as the presencing of the present.

Kristeva's radical heterogeneity is not the same as contradictoriness (moreover even though she uses the notion of "contradiction", it is unclear how it fits within the terms of her theorizing). Here we come to the fundamental problem with the spatial depiction, namely that Kristeva must argue that the unconscious, the (m)Other of the *chora*, always functions synchronically around (and intrusively upon) the symbolic order's domain of signification. This metaphysical assumption, necessary to the idea that the *chora* is a receptacle outside of the conscious discourse of representationality, yet serving to regulate it and even to structure it dispositionally, implies that, whatever the status of the *chora* as epistemologically different from the order of representationality, its meaningfulness intervenes within the unicity of the same time as that of representationality itself. The privilege of the moment as a unity of presencing (exemplified by the signification of "I-now-is") is thus preserved. And this is why the notion of contradictoriness, as contradictoriness inherent to the apparent unity of the moment – a contradictoriness between the semiotic instantiation of the "I-now-is" and that which is within but "otherwise" than semiotic law and order, in both its *sémiotique* and its symbolic variant orderings – cannot be encompassed by the Kristevan interpretation of the dynamic unconscious. Yet it is contradictoriness, as a contradictoriness between temporalities of meaningfulness, that is, I believe, precisely what is exhibited by Freud's discoveries concerning the enunciations of the free-associative subject, the subject of consciousness.

3. Semiosis and the inconceivable "otherwise"

In this paper, we are specifically focused on Freud's discovery of the dynamic unconscious and its implications for the sciences of significatory systems. Thus, we have not been concerned with diverse uses of the term "unconscious" to refer to automatisms and other nonconscious mechanisms of psychological functioning – as reviewed, for example, by Shevrin and Dickman (1980). Rather, we have been more precisely concerned with the semiotics of meaningfulness and with that which disrupts the apparent enclosure and cogency of such meaningfulness. The conclusion to which we are drawn is that Freud's free-associative discovery, from which he advances the notion of the dynamic unconscious, is actually a discovery about consciousness. By attending to the movement of consciousness (exhibited by free-associative discourse as the "I" moves from one construction and communication to the next), it is discovered that consciousness always conceals-reveals, concomitantly and concurrently (in every moment of its instantiation, in every production and reproduction established), something other than what it is manifestly enunciating. And we have concluded here not only that this is a discovery about the inherent composition of consciousness, but also that there are fundamental problems with any spatial depiction or morphological account of this discovery: the dynamic unconscious is not to be considered a storage space for repressed thoughts, feelings or wishes, nor is it to be considered another form of signification signalling to the representationality of consciousness, confusedly and conflictually, as if from afar. I hope that I have shown here, at least preliminarily, that there are insuperable problems (not to mention a substantial ideological mandate to rescue the bankruptcies of the modern era's notion of "science") in any attempt to situate two discrete (but mutually implicated) "spaces" of meaning, or even two discrete (but mutually implicated) orders of signification.

A different mode of interpreting this discovery seems viable. This would be a "reinterpretation" in terms of the composition of consciousness as that of contradictorious temporalities (consciousness as always deferred from itself), and not in terms of congruence or conflict between significatory forms or spaces. This interpretation draws, rather loosely, from the work of Adorno (1966) and Derrida (1967a, 1967b, 1967c, 1972a, 1972b, 1972c), and I elaborate it in my forthcoming book, *Knowing and being since Freud's psychology*. Here I will only point to the main features of this reworking.

I suggest that while consciousness always reveals-conceals something else, the "returning repressed", this does not imply that there is something repressed that is, so to speak, "there", "now", existent in the temporality of the present enunciation but somehow dislocated spatially outside of consciousness, as if exiled to another region but existent in the unity of the same time. That is to say, the dynamic unconscious is not a place of storage for repressed signification; there are not latent thoughts, feelings or wishes, hidden "behind", "beneath" or "beyond" the domain of that which is manifested; and it is misleading to speculate about signification which could be significant yet not signifiable within the domain of consciousness. Rather, I would argue that all signification is "within" this domain actually or potentially available to the "I" of consciousness (which is not to imply that all signification is fully formed, thetic or verbalizable), and that the dynamic unconscious is not "outside" of the semiosis of consciousness but always alienated or estranged within consciousness itself, as the incomprehensible "otherwise" of semiotic law and order. Thus, the ways in which we, as psychoanalysts, are customarily trained to conceive of "conscious/unconscious", under the metaphysical aegis of unity/duality/totality, must be relinquished: the "conscious/unconscious" is not equivalent to the ordinarily conceived relations of culture/nature, figure/ground, surface/depth, text/context, online/offline-processing, literal/figural, or referential/figurative.

Consciousness thinks it knows "what it is talking about" but knows not what it represses – it cannot know what is other than the law and order of its own signification, yet vivacious within its own signification. "All that is" may be significatory, but the mobility of the "I" of enunciation intimates that within its successive constructions and communications something else is at work-play. Even though we can scarcely conceive of this, I suggest that we grasp this "something else" as a temporality that contradicts the unity of the present as manifestation or presencing – contradicts the unified time of semiotic reiterativity, the unicity of representational temporality. The repressed is, to borrow Derrida's terms, under temporal *érasure*; temporally deferred rather than spatially dislocated or morphologically translated into another significatory type or level. It returns incessantly as the revealing-concealing of the "I" and "what it is talking about" – returning as the temporal displacing, dispossessing, deferring, decentering of consciousness with itself. This "returning" is what we call the "dynamics" of the unconscious (and it could be argued here that we might do well to drop the term "unconscious" from our lexicon, since it seems to have an unavoidably situationalistic tone). It is not a transformation (which occurs within a temporal unity), but rather a "transitioning" – the transmutative and truthful character of conscious compositioning as incessantly contradictorious, as an incarnate contradictoriness of temporalities. The returning is this excentricity of the subject of enunciation with itself: the nonidenticality of its presence as presentness or presencing, the nonidenticality of its "I is I" or the "I-now-is" which are its exemplary significations. Thus, the returning is disguisedly expressed. It is a contradictoriness of temporalities eluding the reflective awareness of every moment of construction and communication, every instantiation of consciousness. This "returning" is disguisedly expressed by the *différance* (again to borrow Derrida's terms), the manifestation of signification both as "what it is talking about", the outcome of law and order, and as the trace of something otherwise, something that subverts the law and order by which things appear to be constructed and communicated, appear to hold out the possibility of making sense. In sum, the repressed does not exist in the sense that the form and content of actual or potential signification exists, but it is "as if" rendered inarticulate by temporal *érasure*, its returning as the continual deferral of making sense, of knowing "what I am talking about" – the disruptures, incogitancies and "discontinuities" of what consciousness presents itself to mean and thinks it knows itself to be.

I believe that the revolutionary impetus of Freud's dynamic unconscious is that time is not absolute, not a single linear strand flowing equably, and the present is not a unity of presentness or presencing. Freud exhibited for us, by his method of free-associative discourse, the contradictoriness inherent to the compositioning of consciousness, a discovery that breaks open the apparent unity of the present, intimating the kinesis of an otherwise temporality within the regimentation of semiotic time, intimating the mobility of an incomprehensible "past-future" – to borrow Levinas' term (1947) – disruptively animative but alienated or estranged within the apparent unification of the time of semiotic law and order, the time that is secured by the appearance of the "I-now-is" as if it were identitarian.

The law and order of semiosis requires the unicity of representational time, seemingly, but spuriously, secured for us by the apparent reiterativity of the exemplary signifier "I-now-is" – the signifier of the subject, produced and reproduced by the totality of signification, along with all its circuitry of sender/message/receiver. By "semiosis" I am including here signs of all types and levels, representational and prerepresentational or presentational, symbolic or not, verbal and nonverbal (contrary to Kristeva, I do not grasp the idea of "articulations" or "marks" which are not signs, even if they are not, properly speaking, verbalizable or even re-presentational). The law and order of semiosis requires the unicity of time, time encoded by the apparent reiterativity of representationality. For any sign to signify, whatever its type or level, and however confusedly or conflictually it may do so, it must operate within the unity of a time that privileges presence over absence, identity over difference, and the hierarchy of encoded oppositions over the vitality and kinesis of contradictoriness (cf. Barratt forthcoming). But what psychoanalysis thus shows is that there is a temporality other than the temporality of semiosis; it discovers a mobility that is other than the repetitive constructions and communications of semiotic law and order, the instantiations of an apparently unitary present.

Thus, the "dynamic unconscious" alienated or estranged within consciousness is never a matter of conflict between representations, or even between types and levels of signification, because conflict always presupposes the occurrence of meaningfulness within the selfsame time, the identitarian present. Rather, the dynamic unconscious is the mobility of a contradictoriness that indicts the apparent closure, completion and cogency of semiotic time, the unity of its instantiations of the manifest as present. What Freud discovers is that while everything is indeed signification, there is a temporality other than that of significatory structuration, a temporality disguisedly expressed within the structuration itself. The dynamic unconscious is the other of semiotic law and order, sabotaging the latter's appearances of closure, completion and cogency. Psychoanalysis shows that signification, which always occurs with the appearance of representational time, can never achieve a consciousness that is identical with itself, and can therefore never fully "know" "what it is talking about" – truthfulness will not result from the imperiality of representational production and reproduction.

Elsewhere (under the rubric of "desire"), I have discussed this "otherwise" temporality in terms of the libidinality of the "sexual body" and in terms of the implications of this notion of the dynamic unconscious for the praxis of psychoanalytic discourse (Barratt forthcoming). Here, I wish merely to point to the metaphysical implications of the notion of the dynamic unconscious as the contradictoriness of consciousness and as the "other" of semiosis. The three interpretations I discussed in this paper each miss the radicalism of Freud's discovery because, in a certain sense, they try to conceptualize the incomprehensible and thus to leave unquestioned the metaphysical unicity of time (cf. Derrida 1972a: 29-67; Wood 1989).

The topographic interpretation, for example, depicts an "egological" unconscious – the "I" having the unconscious as its representational "other", a sort of lateral consciousness. The result is that the unconscious stands within the realm of representationality in opposition to the meanings owned by the subject, and is thus able to be appropriated by this subject's expansion of its representational repertoire as a significatory hierarchy of identities and oppositions: all this occurs within the time of representationality, and the notion of contradictoriness remains inconceivable. The Lacanian interpretation dislodges the imperial pretensions of the ego but totalizes semiotic law and order by its notion of the Other such that, again, the unicity of time is assumed and the notion of the subject's contradictoriness remains untouched (the synchronicity of the Other as the totality, and the nugatory quality of the enunciating subject's diachronic movement unto death, both serve these ideological purposes). The Kristevan interpretation of the dynamic unconscious is closer to that advanced in this paper, for the notion of the *chora* is described, at least at certain junctures of Kristeva's writings, as not significatory. It is also not within representationality, and so, being spatially depicted, it gives thinking and speaking a radical heterogeneity. However, this interpretation never does arrive at the notion of an inherent contradictoriness because the unicity of time has not been called into question.

Unlike these interpretations which discuss the subject's "other" as semiotic in one way or another, I believe we have to consider the "other" of semiosis itself. The notion of the psychoanalytic unconscious and the discourse of its discovery suggest the interminable excentricity of consciousness as a locus of contradictoriness within itself, the incessant nonidenticality of its compositioning as movement. Psychoanalysis thus implies that semiosis is indeed "all there is" in life, but that it expresses disguisedly within itself its "other" – the contradictoriness of a temporality that could never be its own, could never be the temporality of the one as the "I" of an apparent identicality. Such an exhibition awkwardly compels us towards a revolution in our notion of what is and is not scientific, because the referentiality and rationality of consciousness is not secureable in the manner that the modern episteme supposed. The discourse of science must now proceed under a postmodernist impetus, aware that a stability of objective or subjective truth is only illusorily attainable.

References

Adorno, Theodor W.

1966 *Negative dialectics*. (Translated by E. B. Ashton.) New York: Seabury, 1973.

Barratt, Barnaby B.

1984 *Psychic reality and psychoanalytic knowing*. Hillsdale NJ: The Analytic Press.

1985 "Psychoanalysis and critique of ideology", *Psychoanalytic Inquiry* 5, 437–470.

1990 "Reawakening the revolution of psychoanalytic method: notes on the human subject, semiosis and desire", *Psychoanalysis and Contemporary Thought* 13, 139–163.

forthcoming *Knowing and being since Freud's psychology*.

Colby, Kenneth M. & Robert J. Stoller

1988 *Cognitive science and psychoanalysis*. Hillsdale NJ: The Analytic Press.

Deleuze, G. & F. Guattari

1972 "Anti-Oedipus", in: *Capitalism and schizophrenia*. Vol. 1. (Translated by R. Hurley, M. Seem & H.R. Lane). Minneapolis MN: University of Minnesota Press, 1983.

Derrida, Jacques

1967a *Of grammatology*. (Translated by G. C. Spivak.) Baltimore MD: Johns Hopkins University Press, 1976.

1967b *Speech and phenomena: and other essays on Husserl's theory of signs*. (Translated by D. B. Allison.) Evanston IL: Northwestern University Press, 1973.

1967c *Writing and difference*. (Translated by A. Bass.) Chicago IL: University of Chicago Press, 1978.

1972a *Margins of philosophy*. (Translated by A. Bass.) Chicago IL: University of Chicago Press, 1982.

1972b *Dissemination*. (Translated by B. Johnson.) Chicago IL: University of Chicago Press, 1981.

1972c *Positions.* (Translated by A. Bass.) Chicago IL: University of Chicago Press, 1981.

Erdelyi, Matthew H.

1985 *Psychoanalysis; Freud's cognitive psychology.* New York: Freeman Press.

Freud, Ernest (ed.)

1960 *Letters of Sigmund Freud.* New York: Basic Books.

Freud, Sigmund

1898 "Zum psychischen Mechanismus der Vergeßlichkeit", G. W. 1, 519–527. London: Imago Publishing Co.

1899 "Über Deckerinnerungen", G.W. 1, 531–554. London: Imago Publishing Co.

1900 *Die Traumdeutung.* G. W. 2-3. London: Imago Publishing Co.

1901 *Zur Psychopathologie des Alltagslebens.* G. W. 4. London: Imago Publishing Co.

1904 "Die Freud'sche psychoanalytische Methode", G. W. 5, 3–10. London: Imago Publishing Co.

1912 "A note on the unconscious in psychoanalysis", S. E. XII, 260–266. London: The Hogarth Press.

1915a "Das Unbewußte", G. W. 10, 264–303. London: Imago Publishing Co.

1915b "Die Verdrängung", G. W. 10, 248–261. London: Imago Publishing Co.

1931 "Letter no. 258, February 7, 1931, to Stefan Zweig", in: Ernest Freud (ed.), 1960, 402–403.

1933 *Neue Folge der Vorlesungen zur Einführung in die Psychoanalyse.* G.W. 15. London: Imago Publishing Co.

Klein, Melanie

1921-63 *The writings of Melanie Klein.* 4 vols. London: Hogarth, 1975.

Kolakowski, Leszek

1968 *Toward a Marxist humanism: essays on the left today.* (Translated by J.Z. Peel.) New York: Grove Press.

Kristeva, Julia

1969 *Séméiotiké: recherches pour une sémanalyse.* Paris: Seuil.

1974 *La révolution du langage poétique.* Paris: Seuil.

1977 *Polylogue.* Paris: Seuil.

1980 *Pouvoirs de l'horreur.* Paris: Seuil.

Lacan, Jacques

1964 *The four fundamental concepts of psychoanalysis.* (Translated by A. Sheridan.) London: Hogarth, 1977.

1977 *Écrits: a selection.* (Translated by A. Sheridan.) London: Tavistock.

1988a *The seminar of Jacques Lacan, book 1: Freud's papers on technique 1953–1954.* (Translated by J. Forrester.) New York: Norton.

1988b *The seminar of Jacques Lacan, book 2: the ego in Freud's theory and in the technique of psychoanalysis 1954–1955.* (Translated by S. Tomaselli.) New York: Norton.

Levinas, Emmanuel

1947 *Time and the other.* (Translated by R.A. Cohen.) Pittsburgh PA: Duquesne University Press, 1987.

Marx, Karl

1844 "Economic and philosophical manuscripts", *Karl Marx, Frederick Engels: collected works.* Vol. 3. New York: International Publishers, 229–346.

Merleau-Ponty, Maurice

1964 *The visible and the invisible.* (Translated by A. Lingis.) Evanston IL: Northwestern University Press, 1968.

Peirce, Charles S.

1931–58 *Collected papers of Charles Sanders Peirce I-VIII.* (Edited by C. Hartshorne & P. Weiss.) Cambridge MA: Harvard University Press, 1988.

Peterfreund, Emanuel

1971 *Information, systems, and psychoanalysis: an evolutionary biological approach to psychoanatic theory.* Psychological Issues VII nos. 1 & 2. New York: International Universities Press.

Plato

1959 *Timaeus* (from Plato's Cosmology). (Translated by F.M. Cornford.) New York: Bobbs.

Rapaport, David

1960 *The structure of psychoanalytic theory: a systematizing attempt.* New York: International Universities Press.

Rorty, Richard (ed.)

1967 *The linguistic turn: recent essays in philosophical method.* Chicago IL: University of Chicago Press.

Saussure, Ferdinand de

1906–11 *Course in general linguistics.* (Translated by W. Baskin.) New York: McGraw Hill, 1966.

Schneiderman, Stuart

1989 "Lacan on Psychoanalysis", paper presented at the meetings of the Division for Psychoanalysis, American Psychological Association, Boston, April 8, 1989.

Shevrin, Howard & Scott Dickman

1980 "The psychological unconscious", *American Psychologist* 35, 421–434.

Wood, David
1989 *The deconstruction of time*. Atlantic Highlands NJ: Humanities Press International.

Freud's "unconscious": a discussion of Barnaby B. Barratt's "Semiosis and its other: notes on the psychoanalytic unconscious"

Michael F. Basch

Barratt argues that Freud's conceptualization of the unconscious as an agency of the mental apparatus separated from, or "below" consciousness, is not a tenable hypothesis. Barratt's criticism of the topographic theory finds me in agreement. Barratt's ultimate solution, as I understand it, seems to be that there is only consciousness, and that what has heretofore been called unconscious in psychoanalysis represents that part of consciousness not at the moment available to itself. How this state of affairs comes about or can be conceptualized is, as Barratt acknowledges, a mystery. I disagree with Barratt's hypothesis as to how we should view what we have been calling the dynamic unconscious. My position would be exactly contrary, namely, that we need not adhere to Freud's concept of a mental apparatus and the topographic division into unconscious, preconscious, and conscious, but that Freud's concept of the unconscious is essentially correct though it did not go far enough. I maintain that all thought, properly speaking, is in the first instance unconscious, and that what is unconscious is not limited to thought content that has been repressed or otherwise defended against. Furthermore, although I fully agree with Barratt's emphasis on the importance of semiotic science for psychoanalysis, what Freud was trying to express with the hypothesis of a mental apparatus has a biological basis.

My argument requires that we go into the history of scientific philosophy so as to understand the problems that Freud, without realizing it, was attempting to resolve with his concept of unconscious thought. The dichotomy between mind and body was established by Rene Descartes (1586–1650) who, in substituting mechanism for animism felt impelled to make an exception for the brain. Prior to Descartes, the activity of living systems had been attributed to the essence, the spirit or *anima*, inherent in the various bodily organs. Descartes, using the recently invented mechanical clock as a metaphor, suggested that the human body could be seen as a collection of interacting parts, and that illness represented a failure of this mechanism which, if the physician was skilled enough, could be repaired as one repaired any other machine. In demystifying the function of the body, Descartes had to make an exception for the brain and the process of thought. The Catholic Church, through the Inquisition, would have severely punished anyone who dared reduce human life to just one more form of animal existence; allowances had to be made for the soul. Accordingly, Descartes suggested that, unlike other organs, the brain became the seat of the soul six weeks after conception when God Almighty, through His grace, instilled a soul into each human being. Henceforth, the involuntary aspects of bodily function were under the control of the brain, but voluntary behavior was under the guidance of the soul, which had taken up residence in the pineal gland. Descartes argued that the evidence for an immortal soul was the presence, in human beings, of reason, consciousness, and thought, all of which were seen to be different facets of this God-given gift. The idea that human beings consist of a body or a soul, later of a body and a mind, left the brain the only animated organ in the body. Although other philosophers raised objections to this idea that thought and consciousness were identical, and that other animals did not reason (Whyte 1960), Descartes' concept won out and is embedded in the very language that we speak today.

Beginning in 1885, Freud, like his teacher Charcot, verified under hypnosis that neurotic symptoms were the consequence of memories of early traumatic events, and that these memories were no longer available to consciousness. Unlike Charcot, Freud did not think of these memories as being less than rational, as the prevailing Cartesian doctrine would have dictated; that is, since reason and consciousness are identical, whatever is not conscious is irrational and not reasoned. Freud recognized as a clinician that the unconscious memories of his patients were far from unreasonable, but, on the contrary, were exquisitely organized; and, as a neurologist, he saw no reason why reason (cerebral activity) and consciousness had to be equated (1888b: 84). Although he apparently was not aware of it, his conclusion was the first systematic challenge to Cartesian mind-body dualism since that first became the received wisdom in the seventeenth century.

Freud did use the term "unconscious" in these early years, but he used it as an adjective, for example, in "Hysteria" where he spoke of "unconscious, automatic cerebral activity" (1888a: 49), "unconscious ideational life" (1888a: 56), and "unconscious ideas" (1888a: 57). In the "Sketches for the 'Preliminary communication' of 1893" (1892a), he evidently had qualms about using the word, clarifying that when he spoke of "unconscious memory" he was referring to the contents of a second state of consciousness (1892a: 150 [see also Freud 1892b-93: 126]), elsewhere called a "restricted" (Freud 1892b-93: 124) or "official" (Breuer & Freud 1893-1895: 76fn) consciousness. As Freud was to point out later, a consciousness of which the individual is not aware raises some serious questions about what the term "consciousness" might then mean (1915: 170), but at this point he had not yet broached that issue.

It is important to recognize at this point that "consciousness" was not itself defined by Freud. He refused to equate it with cerebral activity and remained content to accept it as a phenomenon known to everyone from experience. *Unconscious*, it should be remembered, only means 'not-conscious', at this point, and is, therefore, also only a phenomenological classification.

Freud never had any doubts but that thought was an aspect of brain functioning, and he attempted to create a brain model for thought in his *Project for a scientific psychology* (1895). As I have described elsewhere (Basch 1975), Freud's brain model was based on his study of aphasia (Freud 1891), which had led him to believe that thought was composed of perceptions joined with appropriately descriptive words. He then correlated this hypothesis with his clinical findings on the hypnotic examination of hysterias, in which he found that the traumatic memories or perceptions responsible for the patient's symptoms no longer had available words to describe them. His conception was, therefore, that: (1) hysterias were functional aphasias in which memories had been made unconscious by removing them from verbal expression; and (2) that this process could be reversed by restoring words to the patient with which to describe and examine the memories that had created the patient's difficulties.

At the time that Freud devised the brain model of the *Project for a scientific psychology*, the only force that could account for action was that of energy. As is well known, Freud postulated that the brain was driven by a "psychic energy", which involved the transformation of somatic instincts through a "mysterious leap" into the aforementioned energy, which, when attached to thoughts, would lead to behavior. By blocking the association between memories and words, thought, and ultimately behavior that would produce anxiety and guilt, could be prevented from occurring – this was Freud's explanation for repression. Although this concept of how thought formed, and when necessary could be interdicted, remained with Freud throughout his life, the brain model that he attempted to put together did not satisfy him, and the *Project for a scientific psychology*, or *Psychology for neurologists*, as he originally called it, was not published during his lifetime. Instead, Freud, in the famous chapter VII of *The interpretation of dreams* (1900), postulated a "mental apparatus". He was very clear then and throughout his life that this was a temporary construct to be replaced by a scientifically valid brain model as soon as feasible. It was the original mental apparatus which was composed of the various agencies – unconscious, preconscious, and perception/consciousness. Although Freud, in his model of the mental apparatus, retained the concept of an unconscious and, indeed, reified it, raising it from an adjective to a noun and creating an imaginary spatial realm in which unconscious thoughts took place, by creating the agency perception/consciousness and suggesting that consciousness was the pathway to action (a position he had already taken in the *Project for a scientific psychology*), Freud reinstituted the Cartesian dichotomy that he had done so much to vitiate. In Freud's model of 1900, consciousness, once again, takes the paramount position and, although it is not equated with reason, it is the gateway to action and the final arbiter of behavior. Here Freud was inconsistent with his own discovery that whatever can be accomplished through consciousness can be accomplished without consciousness.

Given the implicit importance of consciousness in Freud's 1900 model, Barratt is quite correct in reaching the conclusion that Freud's topographic unconscious is not a valid concept. However, scientific discoveries made since Freud's time enable us now to formulate a brain model of the sort that Freud was looking for, in which unconscious takes its proper place, and demonstrates the truth of Freud's dictum: whatever can be done with consciousness, can, in principle, be done without it.

With the discovery that information is a quantifiable form of power, and that the generation of information from environmental signals is the capacity that differentiates animate from inanimate, a new era in science was born (Campbell 1982). The brain is an information generating and processing rather than, as Freud believed, an energy processing organ. Indeed, the reception of signals, their transformation into meaningful information, and the use of that information to determine the behavior of the cell, organ, or system is the basis of all purposeful activity and the essence of life. It is also now known, and has been experimentally verified, that the brain's hundred billion cells, each one connected to sixty-thousand or more of its fellows, create a computing organization that generates trillions of bits of information per second. In consciousness, we can process somewhere between twenty to one hundred bits of information per second. Furthermore, it has been experimentally demonstrated that there is a small, but very significant delay between the activity of the brain as it: (1) first organizes signals into perceptions; then (2) compares them with previous experience to see where these perceptions fit; and (3) formulates a response; and only then may make this complex conscious in selected cases. In other words, everything that occurs in the brain is in the first instance unconscious, and a very small portion of brain activity becomes conscious.

We must now qualify what is to be meant by "conscious". Freud always used the term to mean self-conscious, or subjectively aware – knowing that I know, which is what Leibnitz called "apperception". This is important because we know that there is a consciousness of self which is possessed by other animals who are never aware of themselves as objects of their own awareness, as well as by human infants before reflection and the concept of self as such is a possibility for them. For example, when a cat jumps for a mouse some distance away, the cat does not jump to where the mouse is when spied, but to a point ahead of its prey's initial position. The cat possesses, therefore, a sense of self vis-à-vis an external object that permits it to plan its trajectory. Similarly, human infants, long before they can think conceptually, have a sense of self that permits them to behave in ways that clearly indicate that they are aware of their boundaries, both when active and inactive, which enables them to carry out purposeful behavior (Stern 1985).

We must realize, then, that when Freud was talking about the unconscious, he was talking about all brain activity, not only that which had been repressed and defended against. As Kohut and Seitz (1963) pointed out, there is a large area of the dynamic but not defended unconscious which is potentially accessible to consciousness. Furthermore, the delay between perception and self-consciousness allows ample time for the defensive maneuvers which Freud postulated that prevent, in the case of repression, memories from reaching self-consciousness, though these patterns of expectation remain active in the "un-self-conscious".

It is my hypothesis that the purpose of self-consciousness is to permit an individual to replay events that do not fit previously established patterns and are, in one or another way, problematic for the organism. Replaying them in self-consciousness and subjecting these events to the further pattern matching activities of the brain gives that organ the opportunity to deal with them either creatively or dismiss them (Basch 1988). When a particular event is seen as potentially anxiety provoking, and is defended against, the path to self-consciousness is blocked. The result is that the particular anxiety provoking event is no longer subject to the necessary reflection and replay that might permit it to be integrated into the mature problem-solving activity of the brain. This is in keeping with Freud's clinical findings that repressed material operates and draws its strength from the fact that it remains on the early, primitive level of ideation, and has not been subjected to the more mature deliberations and problem-solving activities of later years.

I would agree with Barratt if he postulated only that the psychoanalytic method is a semiotic activity. Indeed, since all of life at every level depends on the generation of information from signals and the appropriate feedback activity that lets that information influence future behavior, all of life is in that respect a semiotic activity. However, the flaws in Freud's explanatory theory, his metapsychology, will not be resolved by transforming "mind" or soul into semiosis. Mind is an aspect of brain functioning, and, therefore, psychology is an aspect of biology that can be studied as can any other organ function. Although Freud's concept of an unconscious in the spatial sense has to be reformulated, the modern-day studies of the brain and information processing corroborate his prescient insight into the nature of thought as primarily non-conscious, and the recognition, although we must not underestimate it because it is the only access we have, that consciousness is at best only a window to the larger realm in which thought activity takes place.

References

Anthony, E. James & Therese Benedek (eds.)
1975 *Depression and human existence.* Boston MA: Little, Brown & Co.
Basch, Michael F.
1975 "Toward a theory that encompasses depression: a revision of existing causal hypotheses in psychoanalysis",in: E. J. Anthony & T. Benedek (eds.), 485–534.
1988 *Understanding psychotherapy: the science behind the art.* New York: Basic Books.
Breuer, Josef & Sigmund Freud
1893–95 *Studies on hysteria.* S.E. II. London: The Hogarth Press.
Campbell, Jeremy
1982 *Grammatical man.* New York: Simon & Schuster.
Freud, Sigmund
1888a "Hysteria", S.E. I, 141–57. London: The Hogarth Press.
1888b "Preface to the translation of Bernheim's *Suggestion* ", S.E. I, 75–87. London: The Hogarth Press.
1891 *On aphasia.* (Translated by E. Stengel.) New York: International Universities Press, 1953.
1892a "Sketches for the 'Preliminary communication of 1893'", S.E. I, 147–154. London: The Hogarth Press.
1892b–93 "A case of successful treatment by hypnotism", S.E. I, 117–128. London: The Hogarth Press.
1895 *Project for a scientific psychology.* S.E. I, 281–397. London: The Hogarth Press.
1900 *The interpretation of dreams.* S.E. IV & V. London: The Hogarth Press.
1915 "The unconscious", S.E. XIV, 159–204. London: The Hogarth Press.
Kohut, Heinz & Philip Seitz
1963 "Concepts and theories of psychoanalysis", in: J. M. Wepman & Ralph Heine (eds.), 113–141.
Stern, Daniel N.
1985 *The interpersonal world of the infant.* New York: Basic Books.
Wepman, J.M. & Ralph Heine (eds.)
1963 *Concepts of personality.* Chicago IL: Aldine.
Whyte, L.L.
1960 *The unconscious before Freud.* New York: Basic Books.

Peirce's notion of abduction and psychoanalytic interpretation [1]

Matthias Kettner

Introduction

Can there be a comprehensive logic of science, a logic of science which would deal both with the methodologies championed in the natural sciences and with those found in the cultural or social sciences? Peirce was an ardent seeker of such a comprehensive logic of science.

In a comprehensive logic of science, Peirce thought, a prominent place would have to be accorded to what he came to call *abduction*, a mode of reasoning not captured by the inductive-deductive dichotomy as traditionally understood. It took a long time for Peirce's seminal ideas about abduction to be appreciated. With the waning of the once widespread belief that the hypothetico-deductive account of scientific reasoning exhausted most of what was logically interesting about science, Peirce's pragmatic notion of scientific inquiry and Peirce's concept of abduction as reasonable hypothesis-formation made their late but momentous impact. In a series of papers starting in 1958, Norwood Russell Hanson revived the quest for an abductive "logic of scientific discovery". The debate which ensued over Hanson's revival of Peircean ideas has served to bring out many difficulties which beset Peirce's concept of abduction. It has, however, also underlined the epistemic relevance of that concept in the philosophy of the natural sciences (Hanson 1958; Gutting 1973; Harris & Hoover 1980; Nickles 1987).

In what follows I suggest that an account of abduction along Peircean lines can provide the centerpiece of a methodology of hermeneutic method and thus can figure prominently in a comprehensive logic of science able to include the cultural sciences. However, I will only have space to argue here for that general point by taking psychoanalysis as my example of a cultural science. I will start off by discussing Peirce's concept of abduction (1.); the aim of this discussion will be to introduce a concept of generalized Peircean abduction and to highlight its connection with hermeneutic methodology (2.). I will then outline the role of *generalized Peircean abduction* in psychoanalysis (3.); finally, I will show how an abduction account of psychoanalytic interpretation can meet an important charge made by Adolf Grünbaum in his philosophical critique of the foundations of psychoanalysis (4.).

1. Peirce's concept of abduction

How can we intelligently look for that of which we are as yet ignorant? How do we rationally conjure up plausible new ideas in the face of problems which challenge our orthodox habits and expectations? These are the leading questions which fuel Peirce's various and somewhat divergent attempts at spelling out the rationality of hypothesis formation in the sciences (Burks 1946; Frankfurt 1958; Fann 1970).

According to Peirce, hypothesis formation in the sciences proceeds by way of a logically distinct mode of inference which Peirce calls abduction: "All the ideas of science come to it by way of abduction. Abduction consists in studying facts and devising a theory to explain them (5.145) ... Abduction is the process of forming explanatory hypotheses. It is the only logical operation which introduces any new idea" (5.172).[2] But what is the relationship between the facts to be studied and an explanatory theory or hypothesis to be devised or accepted on probation? Are there logically interesting differences between, on the one hand, devising or accepting on probation some explanatory hypothesis and confirming or testing it? And what is the scope of the originative character of abduction which Peirce emphasizes so much? If abduction is an inference, what is its canonical logical form and how is it logically warranted? I will address these questions as I go along, starting with Peirce's specification of the canonical logical form of abduction and then pointing out some of its weaknesses. The point of the discussion will be to outline a refined concept of generalized Peircean abduction.

The logical form of abduction, Peirce says, can be represented by the following schema of two premises and conclusion:

> The surprising fact, C, is observed
> But if A were true, C would be a matter of course
> Hence, there is reason to suspect that A is true (5.189).

a) The gist of abduction, then, seems to consist in inferring the reasonableness of an hypothesis A (or henceforth: H) from its ability to incorporate facts which we found surprising into that which we rationally ought to expect. Let us call this the surprise-formula of abduction. Note, first, that according to the surprise-formula, it is not the conceptual content of the hypothesis H, nor H's being true, that is inferred. Rather, what is being inferred is a *plausibility warrrant* for H. The content of H must already be present in the second premise. So if H is a new idea, and if supposedly we get new ideas by abduction, the surprise-formula of abduction fails to represent how these originate. What it does bring out, however, is a conceptual link in rational processes between the emergence of novelty and the demand for a *prima facie* justified account of it. It captures the kind of reason-giving that would ensue if a proponent of a would-be hypothesis were discursively challenged to defend the plausibility of his or her suggestion. For such a challenge to control the outcome of thinking no actual discourse is necessary; merely the capacity of a self-critical thinker to anticipate it is required. The surprise-formula, then, can be taken to represent a regulative idea, either operative in the imaginative processes at the intuitive end of hypothesis invention, by intrinsically constraining such invention, or operative on imaginable hypotheses already at hand by constraining rational choice among them. The surprise-formula is indifferent as to whether explanations get introduced into the realm of the reasonable by selective-eliminative procedure among explanation candidates or by genuinely cooking them up from hitherto non-explicit potentially explanatory resources.

b) What is the logical standing of the surprise-formula? Taken as a purely formal principle, abduction does not seem to be a valid inference because any hypothesis H meeting the demand expressed in the problematic second premise would then allow the inference that H is reasonable. But this would be absurd, as we can see from the following example. Let the surprising fact be that a letter, which I presumed to have put on my hotel room table the other day, has disappeared from the table. On purely formal grounds, the following three thoughts will indistinguishably satisfy the abductive schema:

i. that I must have inadvertently swept if off the table;
ii. that someone from the hotel purloined the letter;
iii. that the letter underwent spontaneous combustion last night.

From each of these three thoughts, and in fact from a million others, if true, my letter's absence from where I had previously placed it would deductively follow and would thus be made a "matter of course". But obviously, assuming normal background conditions, only the first abduced explanation (that I must have inadvertently swept the letter off the table) can be considered reasonable, whereas the second (that someone from the hotel purloined the letter) and third are a far cry from being reasonable. Of course, by varying the relevant background conditions we can think of possible worlds in which it would be a thoroughly reasonable first guess to abductively infer a theft or, more exotic, spontaneous combustion. However, that reasonableness is relative to relevant background conditions at all demonstrates that the validity of abduction depends on an ability to specify background assumptions relevant for the *explanandum* at hand. Such assumptions can be required by a formal principle but they are not themselves formal principles. Hence, a refined notion of generalized Peircean abduction will have to include (1) material background assumptions such that different background assumptions differ in the plausibility ordering which they impose on the infinite space of logically possible explanations.

Peirce himself occasionally emphasized the dependence of abduction on a set of constraints regulating the choice of an explanatory hypothesis. One such principle which Peirce defends on *a priori* grounds is (2) that we must not frame hypotheses which will subsequently block or even stop inquiry. Another constraint on generalized Peircean abduction stems directly from Peirce's *pragmatic principle*: (3) our hypotheses must have pragmatic meaning; i.e., they must admit of being made evidentially sensitive to observations bearing on their content. Plainly, then they must be open to suitable empirical confirmation. Finally, Peirce included (4) considerations of scientific economy (e.g., verificational costs, theoretical fertility) to constrain abduction. Generalized Peircean abduction, then, can validly operate only against a background of normalcy expectations and constraints which Peirce's logical form of abduction fails to represent. Let us now briefly consider and amend another but related weakness of the surprise-formula.

c) Abduction, according to the surprise-formula, looks very much like an inference that is directly data-driven, from problem to explanatory conjecture. However, notwithstanding Peirce's nice metaphor, the facts by themselves do not at all "suggest an explanation". Rather, mere surprising facts hopelessly underdetermine suggestible explanations. Instead of misleadingly construing abduction as an inference from data to explanatory conjecture, then, we should conceive of generalized Peircean abduction as an inference from phenomena plus given explanatory resources (e.g., theories) to corrected variants of such resources under the guidance of discrepant facts (cf. Blachowicz 1987). The pragmatic point of abduction does not so much consist in the creation of novelty for novelty's sake but in the preservation of coherence.[3] Discrepant facts strain explanatory resources which have proved fairly reliable so far but now have to be accommodated to new facts in order to recover overall coherence. Generalized Peircean abduction, I suggest, represents such accommodation by inference to the most natural coherence-saving explanation. What will count as "most natural" will, of course, depend on features of the surprising fact and on the precise aspect under which it is found to be surprising. They will determine (or help to determine) which explanatory resources we should suitably tap, and these in turn will determine (or help to determine) *material principles of coherence* (i.e., principles stronger than logical consistency) and *standards of evaluation for coherence saving*. Let us call this feature of abduction its *domain specificity*.

The domain specificity of abduction is what distinguishes abduction from formal logical principles (which hold in all possible worlds) and what distinguishes the interpretative processes of, for example, an astronomer, a detective or a psychoanalyst, although all three abductively infer explanatory hypotheses (cf. Sebeok

& Sebeok 1979). Thus, Kepler's astronomical abduction that Jupiter's orbit might be of the noncircular type employed other material principles of coherence and other standards of evaluation for coherence saving than, say, a police inspector guessing his way through *The murder in the Rue Morgue.* Freud's psychological abduction that neurotic symptoms may be conflicting expressions of unconscious phantasies evidence material principles of coherence and standards for coherence saving that differ from those of my pedestrian abduction that my letter (in the above example) may have accidentally been swept to the ground.

2. Generalized Peircean abduction and hermeneutic methodology

I want to outline briefly the relevance of generalized Peircean abduction to a comprehensive logic of science that would deal with methodologies championed in the natural sciences as well as with those found in the social sciences, without reductively assimilating social sciences to natural sciences.

From the domain specificity of generalized Peircean abduction it follows that generalized Peircean abduction is relevant to any rational activity aiming at explanation. Generalized Peircean abduction does not privilege some particular kind of *explanans* or *explanandum.* For those who could claim, for example, that the only genuine form of explanation is deduction from laws of physical nature plus initial conditions, no support can be drawn from generalized Peircean abduction. For all the difference that exists between the explanatory resources available in different domains, generalized Peircean abduction works in the domain of everyday action-explanation no less than in the domain of physics or, say, of neurophysiology. Traditionally, contrasts between the so-called natural sciences and the social or moral sciences have been wildly exaggerated. Hackneyed dichotomies such as "understanding versus explaining" or, more recently, "reasons versus causes" are now happily going out of business.

One methodologically important contrast, however, has emerged which proves quite helpful for grouping together large sectors within the social sciences and setting them over against the rest of science. This is the contrast between hermeneutic and non-hermeneutic methods of data assessment. There are a number of important distinctions to be drawn between these two methods which, unfortunately, I cannot explore in this paper. Some clear-cut examples of the contrast I have in mind, therefore, will have to do: compare statistical macroeconomics, on the one hand, and discourse analysis, on the other; or contrast genetic screening and Rorschach testing. Hermeneutics deals with inferring meanings and meaning connections. To the extent that inferable meanings and meaning connections figure in the specification of certain kinds of *explanans* vis-à-vis suitable *explananda*, hermeneutics can be part and parcel of an explanatory enterprise.

We can envision two potential contributions of general Peircean abduction to a comprehensive philosophy of science. Inferring meanings and meaning connections has often been belittled as a purely intuitive, logically uninteresting or, even more damning, rationally unconstrained activity. In this regard, it is interesting to note how many anti-hermeneutic attacks on the methodological credentials of "the operation called *Verstehen*" (Abel 1953) echo logical positivism's misgivings about the alleged rationality of discovery. Nevertheless, a good deal of the business of hermeneutics can be shown to conform to generalized Peircean abduction. By employing a generalized Peircean abduction framework for analytic purposes, interpretation as the ascription of meanings to some text or text-analogue can be seen as a rational activity prompted by surprising discrepancies, constrained by relevant background assumptions, geared to knowledge about relevant explanatory resources in terms of meaning, and directed at rendering surprising facts a matter of course. Thus, the first contribution of generalized Peircean abduction is a general one: generalized Peircean abduction can help us to account for interpretive explanation generally.

A second major contribution of generalized Peircean abduction concerns specifically the explanation of a broad range of human behavior, owing to the fact that human beings are interpretants; that is, they themselves possess and exercise certain abductive capacities and act accordingly. For those inferring them, meanings are not causally ineffective. By specifying abductive capacities and dispositions and by attributing them to some person S, we can predict and explain that portion of the person's behavior in which inferred meanings play a causal role. This pattern of everyday explanation, *explanation by abductive sets*, in fact permeates our everyday interactions. If Peirce was right in describing perceptual judgements as abductions, the explanatory relevance of abductive sets goes right down even to the level of the perceptual behavior we expect people to exhibit; e.g., when we reasonably expect that someone will come to believe that a telephone is ringing upon hearing a telephone ring. Thus, generalized Peircean abduction can make a second contribution to the philosophy of science by providing the centerpiece for an account of interpretative explanation of self-interpreters.

3. The role of generalized Peircean abduction in psychoanalysis

Let us now look specifically at psychoanalysis and what generalized Peircean abduction can do for it. In what follows I take the hackneyed distinction of the clinical and the metapsychological on which many philosophical discussions of psychoanalysis thrive to be of secondary importance because Freud believed: 1) the clinical practice of psychoanalysis to be but one application of the interpretative method, specifically, to benefit neurotic patients; and 2) metapsychology to be a theory which would explain how that method can in fact successfully be so applied.

The methodological core of psychoanalysis is psychoanalytic interpretation. Unfortunately, many psychoanalysts have fallen prey to a comfortable intuitionist rhetoric which depicts their interpretative business as simply "listening with the third ear". Putting aside the narcissistic gains of having a third ear where others have only two, this rhetoric is detrimental to the rational credentials of psychoanalysis. Anybody who studies consensus-formation practices within the profession, especially evident in analyses of "control cases" and their supervision, will notice that psychoanalysts' interpretations, far from being intramentally insulated, are susceptible to rational criticism right from the start (Fleming & Benedek 1966; Thomä & Houben 1967; Kluwer 1970, 1971; Hess 1980; Kettner & Schultz 1985). Psychoanalytic interpretations are proposed on grounds which can be intersubjectively evaluated and criticized. By employing a generalized Peircean abduction framework, patterns of discovery could be discerned and rational criticism of such patterns could be extended to and supplemented by external experts, thus increasing the rational transparency of psychoanalysis' key method. Any attempt to assimilate psychoanalysis to some natural science would be well advised first to take into account the importance which Freud himself attached to the hermeneutic component of the psychoanalytic enterprise. Most metapsychological statements, it is true, make causal claims apparently similar to those made in the natural sciences. Such metapsychological claims (e.g., that paranoia has an homosexual etiology), however, are really high-level abductions generalized in methodologically not very convincing ways from hermeneutically generated low-level abductions. Hermeneutically generated low-level abductions are methodologically at the very foundations of psychoanalysis. And here, analogies with the natural sciences should no longer appear illuminating, because observation-statements in the natural sciences, although being abductions, are not hermeneutically generated abductions.

I realize that the contrast I draw here between hermeneutically generated abductions and abductions generated in non-hermeneutic ways stands badly in need of further elaboration. At least the following points need to be addressed. The input for hermeneutical abduction are data that: 1) admit of being conceived as signs, or sign-analogues, conveying non-natural meaning; 2) are products of human actors; 3) are subject to diachronically operative rules that determine the well- or ill-formedness of such products, which can be judged intersubjectively (Argelander 1981, 1982; Oevermann 1979; Teller & Dahl 1986; Dahl 1988); and 4) can in principle be self-ascribed under action-concepts by their producers (Schafer 1976).

A more sustained look at hermeneutically generated low-level abductions reveals that psychoanalytic interpretations are conceptually continuous with folk-psychology (Malan 1979). That is to say, such interpretations do not type psychological states or episodes in terms of neurophysiological, syntactical, or other flashy "scientific" properties but, rather, in terms of content, specified in the rich intentional vernacular of our commonsense conception of the mental. They do not replace but rather presuppose and extend that conception. When Freud, in his 1915 paper on "The unconscious", rehearsed his reasons for introducing the notion of unconscious yet intentional mental states into psychology, he emphasized that "all the categories which we employ to describe conscious mental acts, such as ideas, purposes, resolutions and so on, can be applied to them ... Thus we shall not hesitate ... to deal with them in the most intimate connection with conscious mental acts" (1915: 168). Other remarks by Freud that can be taken as remarks on abductive rules highlight the conceptual continuity with folk-psychology from a different angle: psychoanalytic interpretations use folk-psychology to exhibit the surprising facts which interpretations have to address and account for. For example:

> If we examine with a critical eye the account that the patient has given us without much trouble or resistance, we shall infallibly discover gaps and imperfections in it ... The train of thought will be visibly interrupted and patched up by the patient as best he may, with a turn of speech or an inadequate explanation; at another point we come upon a motive which would have to be described as a feeble one in a normal person. The patient will not recognize these deficiencies when his attention is drawn to them ... We may make the same demands for logical connection and sufficient motivation in a train of thought, even if it extends into the unconscious, from a hysterical patient as we should from a normal individual (Breuer & Freud 1893-1895: 293).

What, then, does distinguish the meta-abductions of the analyst and the folk-psychological abductions of the person analyzed? What do they purport to explain? Psychoanalytic interpretations do not strive to explain how something works (cf. how the refrigerator maintains a certain low temperature) or how someone manages to do something (cf. how someone memorizes 250 telephone numbers). Rather, psychoanalytic interpretations typically explain why some person, S, does something, A, by ascribing to S's doing A some latent meaning not obvious to S; and by claiming that the latent meaning of S's doing A together with the fact of its not being obvious to S is, or has been, causally relevant for S's doing A (or for the events which constitute S's doing A). How someone manages to do something – for example, to get fired every time when a job begins to demand a high degree of responsibility by starting a quarrel with the boss – can, of course, figure in psychoanalytic interpretations. But such explanations do not constitute interpretations. And although a lot of what Freud has to say about the functioning of the psychic apparatus conforms to the "how does it work" type of question, such hypotheses are not interpretations but pertain to metapsychology.

Psychoanalytic explanations crucially involve reference to idiosyncrasies in someone's making sense of her own behavior; that is, they crucially involve reference to a person's abductive sets. At a high level of abstraction from individual episodes (of persons' exercising their abductive sets), the explanations by abductive sets that psychoanalysts are particularly interested in will usually be found to conform to functional explanation: when all the rich details are dropped from psychoanalytic interpretations, one is typically left with "defense" in order to avoid "hidden feelings" because of the "anxiety" they would create or have created once (cf. Malan's notion of "triangle of defense" and a "triangle of transference" 1979: 79fn).

4. Grünbaum's critique

In the concluding section of my paper, I want to show how an abductive account can meet Adolf Grünbaum's critique of psychoanalytic interpretation, especially Grünbaum's charge of "thematic affinity fallacy". In his powerful attack on the foundations of psychoanalysis, Grünbaum (1984) has claimed, among other things, that the clinical method of psychoanalytic investigation (i.e., the method of free association in therapy) lacks altogether the epistemic resources necessary for validating causal claims about the psychodynamics of unconscious mental states:

> Like Freud, the vast majority of his followers continue to maintain that free associations are crucial for the validation of both their etiologic hypotheses about the causes of neuroses and the psychoanalytic theory of dreams and slips. These advocates cannot dispense with a therapeutic foundation. *For my own part, however, I find it unwarranted to use free association to validate causal inferences* (Grünbaum 1986: 224). [Emphasis added]

Now, for some of Freud's etiological hypotheses linking certain experiences as pathogens (e.g., traumatic experiences) to certain nosological entities (e.g., neuroses), I think that Grünbaum's diagnosis is exactly right, and so is his conclusion, namely that therapy cannot be a self-sufficient research context but has to be supplanted by well designed, extra-clinical studies. Take as an example Freud's case of the Ratman. That a certain experience of the child being punished by his father should have been the "original pathogen" of the Ratman's later compulsory neurosis (that is, the original cause for the onset of the Ratman's rat obsession) is what might be called a *macro-format* etiological hypothesis. Macro-format hypotheses such as Freud's hypothesis concerning the Ratman, if they lend themselves at all to confirmation, surely cannot be confirmed in any strong sense merely by first person recollections of a person's distant past. So far, so good. But Grünbaum overstates his case when he suggests that there is no sound way in which the patient's free associations can be used to validate causal inferences. Associations are used in the clinical setting precisely in order to interpret them. They are used in that way by the analyst and, with the help of the analyst, by the patient, too. Grünbaum's charge, then, suggests that psychoanalytic interpretations in general cannot epistemically live up to the causal claims they contain.

This seems an overly bold claim, and plainly false for the reason that psychoanalytic interpretations are a rather variegated lot. A good deal of the interpretations psychoanalysts give are no more daring as regards their causal import, and no more demanding in what would count as proper validation of their causal import, than much of what passes unproblematically as psychological explanation in everyday life.

There have been many attempts to slice up the domain of interpretations countenanced in therapy along various dimensions (cf. Cheshire 1975: 34). One such taxonomic suggestion is to distinguish interpretations by increasing dependance on a technical theory for specifying the possible range of latent meaning content, or for the way latent meaning content is inferred, or both. Let us contrast two examples, one interpretation being very close to well entrenched folk-psychology, the other being quite technical.

Interpretation 1: Joe's solicitude for his father's welfare is a reaction-formation against Oedipal jealousy.
Interpretation 2: Joe's laughing at his boss' non-funny jokes at the party expressed subservience.

The question of checking whether or not Joe is really projecting his Oedipal guilt raises special problems that do not arise when we try to find out whether or not Joe's surprising susceptibility to the drab humor of his boss really expressed subservience. Another possible dimension for sorting out interpretations is by increasing situational scope and biographical depth of the interpretations' *interpretandum*: on one end, there are interpretations which identify behavior in the here-and-now situation (especially in the highly charged "transference relationship"), as indications of what kind of thing a patient is anxious about, pleased about, angry about, sad about, trying to achieve, or trying to communicate in the arena of her face-to-face interaction with the therapist; at the opposite and confirmationally far more demanding end of the spectrum, there are interpretations which use particular idiosyncratic features of present behavior as cues to understanding the causal origins, and specific form taken by, the patient's disturbed feelings and actions in general.

In more recent publications, Grünbaum has begun to differentiate psychodynamic hypotheses with regard to their confirmability via the confirmational resources of free association. Grünbaum seems to admit that an "analyst's inference that a particular teenage female patient's low self-esteem – as manifested by her expectation of contempt from him – was caused by her life-long awareness of her father's vilifications of her" could have "much better" evidential warrants than Freud's macro-format etiological hypothesis in the case of the Ratman (Grünbaum 1988: 137; see also Holt 1986: 242–244; and Grünbaum's response, 1986: 276). Grünbaum then goes on to suggest that a line ought to be drawn between evidentially warranted and evidentially unwarranted hypotheses according to whether such hypotheses employ the concept of repression. Note that in the "commonsense" interpretation cited above it is awareness of x, not repression of x, that is taken to have a causal effect. However, I doubt that the concept of repression can serve to draw such a line; the psychoanalytic concept of repression itself is rooted in commonsense ("folk") psychology.

Consequently, I conclude that either Grünbaum will have to refine his charges of confirmational incapacity of the method of free association, or his global charge of confirmational incapacity will carry over to a good deal of our entrenched commonsense practices of psychological action-explanation. But if the canons of inductive confirmation upheld in the natural sciences, when transposed to important practices of psychological action-explanation, can make such practices appear vacuous, then surely those canons cannot be the right sort of canons to be so transposed. Or, one would have to claim that the canons of inductive confirmation which are acknowledged in the natural sciences are the sole underwriter for any and every causal hypothesis concerning whatever domain of phenomena under investigation.

One can doubt the latter assumption without getting into the mess of giving up a uniform meaning of the concept of causality. It is dubitable, however, that the concepts of (1) independently observable occurrences of events and of (2) measurable probabilities of such occurrences, concepts which serve the operationalization of the concept of causality in certain domains, are suitable to be applied to every domain of phenomena. Interpretations refer to intentional phenomena. To illustrate the kind of problems that this raises, consider a simple example: that some subject, S, has an intention i (to do A) is a fact about S which (at least for certain sorts of i) cannot be ascertained by observation of S's behavior. And S's acquiring i cannot (at least not for every i) be treated as the occurrence of an event independent of the account S could give of how S itself thinks it acquired i.

An important lesson that can be drawn from the above discussion is that a classification should be developed which would class any psychoanalytic interpretation according to the confirmational burden which that interpretation incurs as a function of the validational standing of the premises which go into the abduction of the interpretation.

Grünbaum substantiates his criticism of psychoanalytic interpretation by focusing on what he labelled the *fallacy of thematic affinity*. Committing the thematic affinity fallacy, according to Grünbaum, consists in inferring causal links from meaning connections. More precisely, the fallacy consists in: first, interpretatively assigning similar meanings to two *interpretanda*; and then inferring, on the strength of the so-established meaning connection, that (the occurrence of) the (temporally) first *interpretandum* is causally relevant for (the occurrence of) the other *interpretandum*; or inferring that both have a common cause. Grünbaum argues that similarity of meaning alone is neither a necessary nor a sufficient condition for there being underlying causal connections, though, of course, similarity of meaning does not preclude there being such connections. According to Grünbaum, when the analyst observes meaning similarities cropping up in the free-association discourse of a patient, the analyst seems no better off than someone who observed, for example, that Thomas Jefferson and John Adams both died at a strikingly similar time "on the 50th anniversary of the Declaration of Independence, written by Jefferson with the aid of a draft to which Adams had contributed" (Grünbaum 1988: 149). Rich correspondences between the two events "do not attest to the two deaths being causally connected" (Grünbaum 1988: 149). To think otherwise would be to commit the meaning-affinity fallacy.

Although the Jefferson-Adams example seems right, it seriously misrepresents what analysts do when they interpret meaning kinship. In cases where it is the patient who assigns meanings and meaning connections by interpreting his or her experiences, the analyst can safely infer that there is an abductive set operative in the patient's ongoing self-interpretative activity which causes the patient to find them significantly related. The natural history of such sets, the retrospective and prospective scope of their operation, can then be further investigated by the analyst. The analyst need not base causal inferences on the strength of meaning affinities alone, as long as an additional premise is available that meanings and their affinities are causally embedded in interpretative processes belonging to a single causally connected mental life, namely that of the person analyzed. Usually, this premise is available.

The causal embedding may be of the following type: if a person S's experiences E1 (of event e1) and E2 (of event e2) appear to S to share thematic meaning, then there is some abductive set operative in S which causes S to assign some meaning M, such that S assigns M to E1 and also to E2. M is what makes E1 and E2 appear (at least to S) as thematic variants of each other, and M is produced by the abductive sets which govern S's interpretative activity. Thematic affinity as apparent to S across different experiences derives from a common source, namely S's interpretative activity.

Thematic affinity of this type justifies the search for an indirect causal connection between the two meaningful experiences, such that each of them is a partial effect of a shared cause. The shared cause is S's interpretative activity working in certain ways, namely under certain abductive sets. This is not to say that the first event e1 causes the (similar) second event e2, nor that the first experience E1 causes the (similar) experience E2; it is to say, rather, that S's interpretative activity plus S's relevant abductive sets cause S's finding E1 and E2 meaningfully related. Note that this is compatible with Freud's view that a person's later experience can determine the meaning of an earlier experience (*Nachträglichkeit*); for this to be possible, all one has to assume is that S's present interpretative activity operates on experiences of present events as well as on recollections of past events. Furthermore, Freud held the stronger view that a recollection of a past event (that was experienced at t1) can become "traumatic" at t2 (i.e., have symptom-forming causal powers) in virtue of the fact that from S's interpretative activity at t2 derives a thematic affinity between the recollection and some meaningful experience at t2. This latter view depends, of course, on further assumptions about the causal powers that meaningful recollections can have.

There are other cases, however, in which it is the analyst who finds experiences significantly related, experiences which the patient as yet fails to find so related. Usually, the analyst will attribute to the patient an abductive set sufficient to square with his own; then the analyst will abduce unconscious constraints which, if they were effective in the patient, would make the patient's failing to see significant relations a matter of course. Such inferences neither are, nor are meant to be, confirmations. They are abductions to unconsciously operating abductive sets of the patient which explain the patient's selective handling of potential meaning.

Finally, as an illustration of thematic affinities in free-association discourse and a psychoanalytic interpretation based thereon, consider the following example:

> A teacher could not maintain discipline in her classroom and the pupils were often defiantly riotous. Although she understood intellectually by what means she could assert her authority, she was unable to do it. When she once, in an analytic session, spoke of the necessity of self-discipline, some childhood memories emerged showing that she had been for a long time a re-

> bellious and unmanageable child. Her difficulty now is particularly related to her unconscious identification with her pupils (Reik 1964: 133).

The analyst's reasoning in this case could be represented by a pattern of abductive inference based on "thematic affinity". I present two versions of that pattern, both of which I think are valid.

(First version)
Abductive premise: It is surprising that S's (= the woman's) behavior manifests features F1, F2 ... Fn.
Abductive premise: It is unlikely (= not to be expected) that S's behavior should show so many features F1, F2 ... Fn that could derive from M without being so derived.
Abductive conclusion: That M is causally relevant for S's behavior is a reasonable hypothesis.

(Second version)
It is unlikely (= not to be expected) that S's behavior should show so many features F1, F2 ... Fn that are surprising in context C1, but which would be expected in context C2, without C2 being causally involved (e.g., via an effective representation of C2, e.g., via S's memory of C2) in S's behavior in context C1.

5. Conclusion

C.S. Peirce has claimed that abduction is a valid form of inference which permeates human experience. Specifying the nature of this claim, I have argued that Peirce's notion of abduction can provide the centerpiece for a normative theory of interpretation. A normative theory of interpretation is needed in the philosophy of the social or moral sciences in order to justify specific "hermeneutic" methods, i.e., methods for inferring meanings and establishing meaning connections. I discussed some weaknesses in Peirce's formulation of abductive inference in order to introduce the concept of generalized Peircean abduction as inference to the most natural coherence-saving explanation of experiential anomalies. Generalized Peircean abduction operates against a background of normalcy-expectations and under constraints which determine standards of evaluation for coherence saving and determine material principles of coherence. Employing generalized Peircean abduction, I clarified the "hermeneutic component" in Freud's method of free association and showed that giving a psychoanalytic interpretation to S implies ascribing to S certain constraints which govern S's abductive capacities. On these grounds, I sought to refute Adolf Grünbaum's charge that Freud's method can establish meaning connections but cannot establish their causal bearing on human behavior.

Notes

1. An earlier version of this paper was delivered at the Charles Sanders Peirce Sesquicentennial Congress held September 5-10, 1989, at Harvard University, Cambridge, Massachusetts.
2. References citing only volume number, decimal point and paragraph number are to Charles S. Peirce, *Collected Papers, Volumes I-VIII*, edited by Charles Hartshore, Paul Weiss and Arthur Banks, published by Harvard University Press, Cambridge MA.
3. From the perspective of the history of science, preservation of coherence can require breaking with an entrenched paradigm, in Kuhn's sense, and creating a new paradigm; it is not essentially a conservative affair. From the perspective of developmental psychology, abduction should not be confused with Piaget's notion of transduction but may shed some light on Piaget's adaptational categories, the assimilation and accommodation of cognitive schemas.

References

Abel, Theodor
1953 "The operation called *Verstehen* ", in: H. Feigl & M. Brodbeck (eds.), 677–687.
Argelander, Herman
1981 "Was ist eine Deutung?" *Psyche* 35, 999–1005.
1982 "Textstruktur und Interpretation ", *Psyche* 36, 700–725.
Bernstein, Richard J.
1965 *Perspectives on Peirce*. New Haven CT: Yale University Press.
Blachowicz, James
1987 "Discovery as correction", *Synthese* 71, 235–321.
Breuer, Josef & Sigmund Freud
1893–95 *Studies on hysteria*. S.E. II. London: The Hogarth Press
Burks, Arthur W.
1946 "Peirce's theory of abduction", *Philosophy of Science* 13, 301–306.
Cheshire, Neil M.
1975 *The nature of psychodynamic interpretation*. New York: John Wiley & Sons.

Dahl, Hartvig
1988 "Frames of mind", in: H. Dahl, H. Kachele and H. Thomä (eds.), 51–66.
Dahl, Hartvig, Horst Kächele & Helmut Thomä (eds.)
1988 *Psychoanalytic process research strategies*. Berlin: Springer Verlag.
Fann, K.T.
1970 *Peirce's theory of abduction*. The Hague: Martinus Nijhoff.
Feigl, Herbert & May Brodbeck (eds.)
1953 *Readings in the philosophy of science*. New York: Appleton.
Fleming, Joan & Therese Benedek
1983 *Psychoanalytic supervision*. New York: International Universities Press.
Frankfurt, Harry G.
1958 "Peirce's notion of abduction", *Journal of Philosophy* 55, 593–597.
Freud, Sigmund
1915 "The unconscious", S.E. XIV, 159–215. London: The Hogarth Press.
Grünbaum, Adolf
1984 *The foundations of psychoanalysis; a philosophical critique*. Berkeley CA: University of California Press.
1986 "Précis of *The foundation of psychoanalysis; a philosophical critique* ", *The Behavioral and Brain Sciences* 9, 217–228.
1988 "The role of the case study method", in: H. Vetter & L. Nagl (eds.), 134–175.
Gutting, Gary
1973 "A defense of the logic of discovery", *Philosophical Forum* 4, 384–405.
Hanson, Norwood Russell
1958 "The logic of discovery", *Journal of Philosophy* 55(25), 1073–1089.
1965 "Notes toward a logic of discovery", in: R.J. Bernstein (ed.), 42–65.
Harris, James F. & Kevin D. Hoover
1980 "Abduction and the new riddle of induction", *Monist* 63, 329–341.
Hess, Allen K. (ed.)
1980 *Psychotherapy supervision –theory, research and practice*. New York: Wiley and Sons.
Holt, Robert
1986 "Some reflections on testing psychoanalytic hypotheses", *Behavioral and Brain Sciences* 9 (2), 242–244.
Kettner, Matthias & Petra C. Schulz
1985 "Untersuchungen zur Konstitution fokaler Deutungsmuster anhand von Verbatim-Supervisionsprotokollen".[Unpublished Diplom-Thesis, J.W. Goethe-Universität, Frankfurt.]

Malan, David H.
1979 *Individual psychotherapy and the science of psychodynamics.* London: Butterworth.
Nickles, Thomas
1987 "Methodology, heuristics and rationality", in: J.C. Pitt & M. Pera (eds.), 103–132.
Oevermann, Ulrich
1979 "Die Methodologie einer "objektiven Hermeneutik" und ihre allgemeine forschungslogische Bedeutung fur die Sozialwissenschaften", in: H.G. Soeffner (ed.), 352–434.
Peirce, Charles S.
1931–58 *Collected papers* I–VIII. (Edited by C. Hartshorne, P. Weiss & A. Burks.) Cambridge MA: Harvard University Press.
Pitt, Joseph C. & Marcello Pera (eds.)
1987 *Rational changes in science.* Dordrecht: Reidel.
Reik, Theodor
1964 *Voices from the inaudible. the patients speak.* New York: Farrar & Straus.
Schafer, Roy
1976 *A new language for psychoanalysis.* New Haven CT: Yale University Press.
Sebeok, Thomas A. & Jean Umiker-Sebeok
1979 "You know my method: a juxtaposition of Charles S. Peirce and Sherlock Holmes", *Semiotica* 26.
Soeffner, Hans-Georg (ed.)
1979 *Interpretative Verfahren in den Sozial-und Textwissenschaften.* Stuttgart: Metzeler.
Teller, Virginia & Hartvig Dahl
1986 "The microstructure of free association", *Journal of the American Psychoanalytic Association* 34, 763–798.
Thomä, Helmut & Antoon Houben
1967 "Über die Validierung psychoanalytischer Theorien durch die Untersuchung von Deutungsaktionen", *Psyche* 21, 664–692.
Vetter, Helmuth & Ludwig Nagl (eds.)
1988 *Die Philosophen und Freud.* Wien: Oldenbourg.

The case of Frau Doktor K.: a Lacanian psychosis

Bernard Rubin

Introduction

This paper describes the treatment of a patient with a paranoid psychosis whom I began treating 25 years ago. What I want to demonstrate is how some of Lacan's ideas enable me to understand that patient and her illness better than I had in my more traditional, original formulation of her treatment.

I will use three of Lacan's concepts, illustrated with excerpts from my record of treatment and from a lengthy illustrated journal which I received from the patient many years after treatment ended. The three Lacanian concepts are:

i. that a subject is constituted by lack;
ii. that the subject is constituted by her relationship to the signifier, which often carries greater weight than the signified;
iii. that sexual difference can only occur when the subject has moved from the imaginary into the symbolic register by acceptance of the paternal taboo against incest, that is, the father's "no".

How these concepts are used will become clear as I describe the patient, the problem, and the treatment. I should add that I will eventually describe three signifiers central to the patient's discourse, which will clarify Lacanian concepts i and ii above. They are the sound images: [*fence*], [*horse*], and [*blood*]. Subsequently, I will describe how this patient's refusal to be constituted by sexual difference, that is, her inability to accept the father's "no", results in a problematic tension between the symbolic and imaginary registers.

1. Case history

This 60-year-old woman was introduced to me by her husband as suffering from "paranoia querelans". For a week she had been panicked, feeling that she was being followed, and that gas was being introduced through her apartment vents in order to render her unconscious. During that week she had refused to speak to her husband.

She was born in Germany at the turn of this century. I shall call her Frau K. At first sight she was a solid-looking, somewhat carelessly dressed woman of medium height, who wore glasses. Without them she looked like Gertrude Stein. She spoke with a distinct and distinctive German accent, yet would not speak German, even when repeating her favorite expression,"if God shoots a broom." I learned, but not from her, that it was a curious translation of the phrase, "*wenn Gott schütze Rom*" ('if God protect Rome'), usually said ironically by North German Protestants.

She appeared at ease when talking about the past, but became vague and discomfited when asked about details of the week prior to my seeing her. She was suspicious and anxious. She asked to be protected from "them", who were after her and trying to gas her. The implication was that "they" were Nazis, who wanted to control her mind and soul, or kill her. She asked me to have her husband hand-deliver a letter to a South American consulate asking for asylum. When she was asked to specify her problem, she said, "I can tell you about it in three sentences", but then became vague. There did seem to be three disturbing circumstances:

1. She had spoken to the president of a South American country, who was visiting Chicago, and was worried about him.
2. Her apartment was being repainted. She thought that one of the painters acted like a member of the Gestapo. She became so agitated that her husband moved to a nearby hotel. She moved into another room of their apartment, saying, "If he can be comfortable, why can't I?"
3. She thought that she had developed a contact dermatitis from the paint which threatened her with anaphylactic shock. Generally she thought people were acting strangely. She wondered if I was trying to hypnotize her in order to get information. I decided that she was suffering from paranoia with anxiety, paranoid delusions and olfactory hallucinations, and I hospitalized her.

It was not the first time this had happened. In January 1946, when on leave in England from her position as an army physician in India, she suddenly stopped writing to her husband, and when he called, she said she did not want to see him. She later told him that she had hyperthyroidism, but because of anxiety had to be hospitalized. She said that her psychiatrist was "supercilious", and that he tried to make her problem an "hysterical" one. When she returned to India, her husband said that she was different: she argued with everyone; was leftist in her political views; and stopped all sexual contact with him, saying she had heart disease. She appeared depressed, which he attributed to her envy over his professional success.

Frau K. was the firstborn to parents of the landed Junker class in Germany. Her father was 37 at the time of her birth, and her mother was 23. A more favored brother was born one and a half years later. The family lived in a manor house on a farm of thousands of acres. There were servants, farm workers, and governesses for the children's education. Members of the father's family lived nearby and visited; the mother had been adopted and had no siblings.

Frau K. was a strong, active child, who often acted the tomboy. She idealized her father, felt her mother had little or no interest in her, and hated her brother. By the time she was 10 years old, it was clear that her father was in the late stages of syphilis, and he died when she was 14, after dissipating the family properties and money. Frau K. became a vagabond, but had completed Gymnasium and did some teaching in physical education by the time she was 28. At 30 she entered medical school in Vienna, a desire stimulated by her father's physical deterioration. One year later she married her Jewish professor of pathology. He fled Austria in 1938, and she followed after finishing her studies in 1939. They eventually got to India and joined the British Army, where she was a physician in a general hospital until the end of World War II.

Frau K.'s mother and brother were held as minor Nazis by the British Occupation Forces in Germany, and were released through the intervention of her husband. Her brother returned to South America, while her mother joined her in India, but quickly went on to South America because of their quarreling. Frau K. was successful as a dressmaker and breeder of dogs, but both of these endeavors came to little because of her quarreling. Increasingly dissatisfied, she got visas to the United States and her husband agreed to emigrate with her.

Unfortunately, Frau K. immediately equated the materialism of this country with that of Nazi Germany. She tried and gave up two medical residencies because of anxiety. Nevertheless, after moving to another east coast city, she began a new career as a painter and sculptor. She taught art at the university and had a very successful show at an important gallery. In 1957 her husband came to Chicago because of a professional opportunity, and she moved with him.

Beginning in 1960 Frau K. began a number of frantic trips to South America to visit her remaining family. Each time she returned she spoke of being followed, of Nazis who worked as porters and pursers on the various ships she had taken. She seemed to quiet down after a few months back home, until the episode that brought us together.

I decided to treat Frau K. with psychotherapy. This was predicated on my understanding, at that time, of notions regarding the psychological defense of projection and its relationship to latent homosexuality as developed by Freud in his 1911 monograph on the Schreber case, "Psycho-analytic notes on an autobiographical account of a case of paranoia (dementia paranoides)". With Frau K., it was as if Schreber, with gender finally changed, had come back to life. Even the timing was similar: a hypochondriacal attack at age 45, and then a second more prolonged psychotic state beginning in her mid-50s. My emphasis in treatment was on her self-esteem, the ambivalence regarding gender, the projections of hatred in the form of delusions of persecution and mind control, and the hallucinations of being gassed.

Frau K. hated men without reservation. "Men are shits", she would say. As an adolescent she had been seduced by some of those to whom she had turned for help. She was obsessed with the belief that she had granuloma inguinale, which she thought was the result of a sexual encounter during her *Wander* years. At the same time, she admired her father's progressive ideas and her husband's intellect. Sarcasm colored her remarks about "ladies" in general, and her mother in particular. She longed to be close to a younger woman whom she might treat as she had wanted to be treated as a child, but she was afraid of being left.

Frau K. was afraid of her husband in this episode of illness. She thought that he wanted to introduce a medicinal substance into her food which would cause her to die. This delusion alternated with feelings of intense loneliness, related in part to her husband's professional life, and his involvement with another woman whom Frau K. called a "Nazi bitch". She added that her husband had been involved with other "Nazi bitches" in India after World War II.

I tried to bolster her self-esteem. She was a marvelous storyteller. She was a good painter, and we discussed her paintings and drawings. Her recurrent concern was with fascism in the world, which she called a "toxic" problem that caused her "allergy". I connected her toxic problem with alienation, compounded by her anger which caused a shift to hypochondriasis. In a short time she left the hospital, and I continued to see her in my office.

She was without symptoms and went back to South America. I received a photo of her from there with a note on the back which stated: "A foolscap has been thrown. If somebody puts it on, it's not my fault." I thought that the message was, 'don't blame me for being dumb again'. Later, I learned that she had quarreled dreadfully with her family; and that she had purchased two cemetery lots, one for her mother and one for herself.

The next year she went to England to visit old friends. I received a card which said:

> Speaking of coincidences. As I sat down to have my photo taken, they played, 'Hang down your head, Tom Dooley; hang down your head, and cry.' I laugh in spite of it. Don't fence me in.

This was typical of her repeated responses to songs with songs, and of her incorporation of some lyrics into her discourse.

Frau K. was intermittently preoccupied with the question of her husband's hatred of her. She often said, "I need it like a hole in the head." That statement could refer to her husband, marriage, psychiatric treatment, or her mental state. She again returned to South America, as it turned out for the last time, to visit her mother, who died a few years later at 92. Thirteen years after her mother's death, Frau K. died, having insisted just before on being buried next to her mother's grave. She died, literally, of a hole in the head: a squamous cell carcinoma of the scalp, which she refused to treat, hiding the ever-enlarging hole with her scarves.

2. The mechanism of paranoia

Lacan's entry to the language of the unconscious was in 1932 with his doctoral thesis, "Paranoid psychosis and its relation to the personality". For the most part he was fascinated by the psychotic's allusions, neologisms and language fragmentation. He argued that psychosis was due to a fixation at the stage of ideal image formation (his o-o' axis). The thesis anticipated his concept of the mirror stage, the child's experiences between 6 and 18 months of age, in which a fragmented self or the primordial "I" begins its journey of alienation from a specular "I" – the "I" modeled on the mirror image, which deceives the child into a belief of wholeness and otherness – to the social "I", the "I" objectified in the dialectic of language. This part of the subject's history, before being constituted within the dialectic of language, is for Lacan the imaginary moment. As in dreams, the imaginary is dominated by homologies and binary extremes, the appearance of doubles and hallucinations. The mother, or to be more exact, a part of her – the breast – is the initial object of the child's desire (*objet petit a*). When threatened with its loss, the signifying activity of the unconscious commences: that is, the child begins to be constituted by his language. This movement from the imaginary to the symbolic register enables the child to function as a subject. The paradigmatic example of the use of language to control loss is the *fort-da* game mentioned by Freud. The two movements of 'gone' (*fort*) and 'here' (*da*) – represented by O-A, [*ooh-aah*], the vowels of *fort-da* are twice mentioned, first in *The interpretation of dreams* (1900) and again in *Beyond the pleasure principle* (1920). These first two phonemes indicate the signifying transaction which allows the child to shift from the loss of the object of its desire to inaugurating its mother's desire as its own. When this particular signifying transaction does not occur, psychosis is the result.

What does it mean to say that psychosis has its roots in the "imaginary", before language has restored the self to its function as subject? Does it mean that for the psychotic there is no "symbolic"? No, for every child is born into language. Rather, it has to do with the absence of a particular symbolic shift, so that tension between the imaginary and symbolic prevents the integration of certain signifiers in the subject's unconscious, with their subsequent appearance in the "real": the realm of symptoms.

For example: It seemed at one point in treatment that Frau K. might be more comfortable speaking German, and I told her to do so if she wished. She responded angrily, "*Ich habe Es vergessen.*" ('I have forgotten it'.) *Es*, of course, is her referent to the German language, but 'it' also refers to the unconscious, *das Es* of Freud. This distinction between the conscious or signified, and the unconscious or signifier, is for Lacan the unfolding of the Freudian systems, "preconscious/ unconscious". However, unlike Freud, for Lacan the dividing line between these two systems is one that can be crossed as the subject goes back to where he was an unconscious. It is only in that way that, for Lacan, Freud's dictum, *Wo Es war, soll Ich werden*, ('Where It was, I shall become') makes any sense. Lacan elaborates this dictum: "There where it was just now, there where it was for a while, between the extinction that is still glowing and a birth that is retarded, "I" can come into being and disappear from what I say" (1977: 300). For the subject to be there where "it" was, there must be a shift between the elementary signifiers into the unconscious (pre-conscious/unconscious). To help explain the antithesis between Frau K.'s *Ich habe Es vergessen* and *Wo Es war, soll Ich werden* I return to Lacan, who himself returns to Freud and the Schreber case.

In Lacan's study of the Schreber case, "On the question preliminary to any possible treatment of psychosis" (1977: 179–225), he found that in the subject (Schreber), signifiers that would ordinarily be closed, that is, repressed, are represented. Lacan searched, in Freud, for a defense mechanism specific to psychosis and related to projection. After all, Freud had promised twice (1911: 66;71) to elucidate fully the defense of projection, but did not. Instead, he used the word *Verwerfung*, which Lacan calls 'foreclosure' (*foreclusion*). According to Lacan, this follows Freud's much earlier notion of a defense mechanism that is distinct from repression, related to projection, and specific to psychosis. Freud notes in the Schreber case: "It is incorrect to say that the perception that was supressed internally is projected outward; the truth, is rather, as we now see, that what was abolished internally returns from without" (1911: 71).

Verwerfung is that something which is not symbolized, but which ought to be. The foreclosed signifiers are not integrated into the subject's unconscious; they do not return from the inside, but re-emerge in the "real" through hallucination. Foreclosure expresses itself by: 1) a withdrawal of cathexis from the external world; and 2) a loss of reality related to the primary mechanism of separation from, and expulsion of, intolerable perceptions.

As an example, I offer the following telephone conversation which occurred several times between the patient and me:

Frau K.: "Did you just call me?"
R: "No, is something wrong?"
Frau K.: "Stop calling me! I have been trying to go to the bathroom, and your calls are making me constipated."

For Lacan this would represent an accident in the symbolic register: the foreclosure of the paternal metaphor "no" in place of the other. This deficit of the symbolic gives psychosis its essential character. For a psychosis to be triggered later in life, as with Schreber and Frau K., the paternal authority being foreclosed must come again into opposition to the subject. Thus, the hallucinated ringing of the phone returns in opposition to the subject's desire to defecate. We shall see later how bowel movements were connected by Frau K. with paternal authority.

3. Attempts at interpretation

Some years after my treatment of Frau K. had ended, she gave me a lengthy illustrated journal entitled, "The first part of my life – for better understanding", whose text and accompanying illustrations provided examples of her use of language to demonstrate what might be called a Lacanian psychosis.[1] Frau K.'s discourse was enmeshed in curious relationships between German and English words, song titles and lyrics, and quotations from a number of other sources. As an illustration of her language "breakdown", I will examine the way in which three signifiers – *fence, horse*, and *blood* – appeared in her psychotherapy and journal.

The first, *fence*, she often alluded to in the song title, "Don't fence me in." The following excerpts from Frau K.'s journal, presented chronologically, represent a fence-like structure, or the function of fencing off.

> "When I was born it was winter and bitterly cold. Six rooms parted me from the inhabited world."
> "We were tied to our *Gitterbetts* (literally a 'fence-bed', i.e., a crib)."
> "I was in my playpen – a horrible jail."
> "I had to live with the world outside of me, and always bumped my head against it."
> "When I was ten my mother thought I was *verwachsen* ('deformed'). In the torture chamber of the doctor I was put in these contraptions. There was no way out. Don't fence me in!"
> "Nobody could hold me. My father said, *Reisende Leute soll man nicht aufhalten* ('one should not impede traveling persons')."

"I had nightmares of flying, defying gravity, leaving the earth, and then crashing."
"I glanced at our burial place. Surrounded by a fence. Why a fence? There was no escape, but for ghosts. No, I didn't want to be buried there even if it was our place, it was so cold and dark there, so desperately lonely."

Fence can signify emptiness, inside, outside, crib, playpen, any room, office, torture chamber, jail, mother earth, an estate, and the family "plot" in both senses of the word. Signifieds proliferate, but the constant (unconscious) meaning is to be parted from, or to be held within or back. Fences lead to a state of emptiness, to panic; for Frau K. they are unnatural.

Therefore the fence is a metaphor for that which imprisons Frau K. in an empty, impenetrable space, where her words echo and become distorted. The space is her psyche, but meaning can only be experienced as outside of it.

The second signifier is *horse*. The following are excerpts from Frau K.'s journal indicating her passion for and identification with horses:

"I started very young, clinging to my toy horse."
"Before my pony I rode everything – even a pig."
"I had dream horses, one black named Nati, and one white named Ali. I rode them in my *Gitterbett* (a metaphor for masturbation, as she was told by her mother that she was tied to her crib in order to prevent her from doing bad things)."
"They became I and I became them. My dreams were my reality."
"My grandmother spotted it first. She said, *Etwas muß geschehen, das Kind ist ja ganz Pferd* ('Something must be done, the child is really all horse')."
"I was a dark horse always, the unknown entity."
"My father had a wild Hungarian stallion. He could not break him so he shot him."
"Wotan rode with wild horses, bringing death."

Frau K. fused with the phallus as part-object. There is no distinction between the specular "I" and some part of the other (Lacan 1977: 1–7). The danger of being the horse, the phallus, is that it brings death, or even is Death.

Frau K. identified with her father, but only with that part which represented power, his phallus. This identification was a perception never internalized, but existing like a false reflection of herself in a mirror, and confused with her own body image. Her power, her phallus, was her words, uttered with anger and contempt at her auditor. Yet, it was often that she was herself the auditor of these words, directed back to her as auditory hallucinations.

The third signifier is *blood* which has a temporal and literal connection with the following phrases:

> "Everything is finally the same, rot and decay."
> "I need it like a hole in the head."
> "Where it finally ends up, is that the bottom?"

How these statements are related to, as well as amplify, the meaning of the signifier *blood* will become apparent as we read the following excerpts from Frau K.'s treatment with me and her journal:

> "My father is a God, and the Gods cannot be portrayed." (This statement is illustrated by an empty picture frame.)
> "My father's grandfather, his father, and he all had syphilis. Father developed progressive paralysis, and I lost him when I was 14. He died in a disgusting and rotten way. But the most disgusting thing was my mother's pretending, lying and hiding."
> "I remember when they took my W.R. (Wasserman test), and the blood ran over my white sailor suit." (A metaphor for menstruation.)
> "When I was 10 my cousin Elisabeth asked me: *Spricht denn nicht in Dir die Stimme des Bluts?* ('Doesn't the voice of your blood – your patrimony – speak in you') I said: What is that, I hear nothing."
> "A year later, when they locked him up, the dirty secret of his illness fell like a dark veil over my already dark childhood. I discovered Nietzsche, who then became my God, my father."
> "I encountered death early in life: a chicken with its head cut off, runs for dear life; a little girl in our village spitting blood, and I saw Death on a horse riding through the village; a neighbor bleeding his life away through his mouth, and a stinking chamber pot under his bed."

The blood comes from the bottom, and is at the bottom of all things:

> "I was terrified of dying. There are many deaths, each leaves you emptier. Like peeling an artichoke, till you get to the bottom. I mean leaf, but it comes to the same."
> "When they sold the estate I was rooted there, and the bottom of my world fell out. I dragged my roots with me the rest of my life."

And then two memories of two chairs:

> "I was held in a chair by the nurse, while the doctor took my adenoids; blood poured from my mouth."
> "It was a chair I was forced to sit in, underneath a terrible contraption that stank. I had to do *ka-ka* and didn't want to."

The passion of her father's blood had led to death, as the passion of her blood, she felt, must do the same. It is the absence of substance itself – blood, feces, the self – like the portrait of her father, an empty frame. Life is a defoliation, a decay, which she tried to retard by carrying along with her a document from Nazi Germany, her *Prufungsergebnis*, which attested to her being *deutschblutig* (of Aryan blood – pure blood). But in the end, blood and feces are the same. The secret, the dirty, disgusting secret of her mother about her father's syphilis becomes Frau K.'s phantom illness – her delusion of having a venereal disease. But it is also an hallucination, for she could see the signs imprinted on her body.[2]

Blood is necessarily her metaphor of life. But the evidence for its existence is when it appears outside, as loss. To see or even sense blood (or feces) exiting the body is a way of knowing one has life, but also knowing that one is in the process of losing it.

> "I was told I nearly died as a baby. I didn't want to drink from my mother. 1–1/2 years later my brother was born; he drank from her plenty."
> "Very early I noticed my baby brother and I were different. He challenged me to a pissing contest. Needless to say I faced utter defeat, but I refused to accept there were things in the world I couldn't get."
> "My mother said I was so stubborn I would grow horns."
> "I was told that little girls were not supposed to study. My intellect was sharp as a razor; it was the only weapon I had."
> "My father said: you are my boy; my brother was always a good solid piece of nothingness."
> "I hated dolls, except one with black hair and brown eyes. It was not a boy, and certainly not a girl. It stood between the sexes as helplessly as I did."
> "I watched animals (coupling), they were beautiful with no strings attached."
> "I saw the afterbirth of a cow. I was frightened and remembered the smell. The smell followed me for years afterward."
> "That line of the devine is not for me (i.e., holy motherhood)."
> "Men would sink to the level of animals, and then surround it with a lie; it disgusted me."
> "I hated the smell of diapers. Holy motherhood, the protective curve of her back over him."
> "I had this terrible dream. I looked down in the hidden lake with its dry,

> sickly whispering, and saw white naked babies, resting in the mud, refusing to disintegrate."
> "I wanted to kill my brother."

And in relation to loving another:

> "Fräulein K. was the first woman in my life that I loved consciously. I loved her with no restrictions; like a dog lying on its back in front of its master."
> "If she went to bed with my father and not with me, even that I could forgive."
> "I think she must have been Jewish, and that would explain a lot in my later years."

Sexual difference is the organizing principle of the symbolic order. Frau K. worked to erode that difference each time it seemed to assert itself, as with the birth of her brother, her feelings about her mother and father, menarche, and the awareness of any sexual passion. That the subject must struggle in defining this difference is central to Lacan's notion that the subject is defined by "lack". In this notion of lack, the ego is the source of the illusion of wholeness, rather than the source of its intactness. As S. Leclaire notes: "The ego is the site of the subject's imaginary identifications" (1958).

Lacan invokes, as did Freud earlier in his *Three essays on the theory of sexuality* (1905) and *Beyond the pleasure principle* (1920), the story told by Aristophanes in Plato's *Symposium* (1973) to explain the lack. Aristophanes tells how the human subject originally was derived from a whole – a quarrelsome, difficult subject with all the parts of what is now male and female. The Gods punished this unitary person by splitting it in half, male sexual organs on one side, female on the other. The existence of these two parts was then dominated by the desire to recover its missing complement. The division is sexual in nature, and can only be resolved by heterosexual union and procreation. Lacan might add to the story of Aristophanes, that the difference also absolutely determines the subject's social identity. But the movement of Frau K. is contrary. That is, it is not toward sexual meaning, her femininity, but rather toward androgynous being: from meaning to being.

For Frau K. gender was a source of confusion. At times she felt like a man trapped in the body of a woman. But more often, she felt like a helpless, genderless child for whom survival was the only issue.

4. Further attempts at interpretation

I had said that I would return to Frau K.'s concern with her bowel movements. As we have seen, her *ka-ka* is peculiarly connected with blood and decay, as well as a concern with her ability to control its loss of destruction. Her initials were K.K., and she wrote her name so that the first letter of her given (chosen) name, and of her married name were significantly larger than the letters that followed. Her family name, F ..., she felt belonged to her mother and brother, not to her. When she spoke her name it was with an explosive emphasis on the first letter of each name. She would say, I am K ... K ...!

For Lacan, as has been amply noted, the unconscious is organized like language. The splitting of the subject results from the fact that she speaks, thus becoming a signifier. As Lacan notes in his further amplification of the Freudian dictum mentioned earlier, "I am what I think, therefore I am": divide the "I am" of existence from the "I am" of meaning. This splitting must be taken as being principle, and as the first outline of repression, which as we know establishes the unconscious" (1966).

This splitting starts with primal repression in which certain phonemes (e.g., the O-A of the *fort-da*) become part of the unconscious as language; in fact, the first signifier as such. In other words, psychical representation of the imaginary instinct sinks into the unconscious under the effect of countercathexis of the elementary phonemes. Now the process of secondary repression can occur, for the fixation of a few key signifiers, consisting of certain paired phonemes, is the foundation, that is, the relative fixity of signifier to signified found in language. Language is then radically excluded from thought, as it enters into it by way of the sign that alienates it.

For Frau K. the paired phonemes, *ka-ka*, unlike O-A, have no opposition. No other is implied, but rather only an aspect of the self. Her journal had stated: "six rooms separated me from the inhabited world." This is a defect of primary repression. In order to examine that defect more carefully, it will be necessary to return to her expression, "if God shoots a broom", and what I am suggesting is its German (original) origin, "*wenn Gott schütze Rom*". The English phrase is remembered, spoken, and the latter forgotten, lost. I think that the likely relationship of the one to the other could be explained by Frau K.'s expletive: "*Ich habe Es vergessen*". The German phrase, the original, must somehow reside in unconscious language, the effect of primal repression, and therefore partakes of the symbolic. The English word is foreclosed (*verwerfen*, Freud), representing a perception abolished internally, returned from without, as a hallucination. Thus the German phrase is an expression of the signifiers of the symbolic, while the English phrase is an expression related to phonemes, never quite repressed, emerging from the imaginary into the real. For Frau K. the tension is between the signifiers and the phonemes, between the symbolic and the imaginary with its consequences of paranoia; that is, symptoms in the real.

Let us now look at both phrases. The first phrase: "if God shoots a broom".

The first word, *God*:

God=father	"My father was a God."
father=Him	"I worshipped him."
Him=Death	"I played cat-and-mouse with Him."
Death=Wotan	"Wotan rode wild horses bringing death."
God=Frau K.	"I played at being God many times in my life."

Therefore, I, the Father, bring Death; to be the father is to be Death. I am Death, the Father – the "dark horse".

The second word, *shoots*:

shoot=subjugate	"We had a black stallion who was Life itself."
	"He refused to be broken."
subjugate=kill	"My father shot him, and it broke my heart."
subjugate=beat	"Father beat me with a stick. It was routine. My victory was to be stronger than Him, not to cry."
	"The beatings were like an Amen in Church, except the next day."

The third word, a *broom*:

broomstick=passion	"The pain I loathed, but the feeling that I defeated Him, I loved. I loved his passion."
passion=horse	"I ride my dream (broomstick) horse to exhaustion."
horse=stick	"When I rode my wild horse, I used to pray: God, let me die at this wonderful moment."

"I was thrown and lost my breath" (speech).

How do we make sense of this? Passion is the stick which men have and women lack. She once said angrily, "To look like a lady, it is as if one had swallowed a stick." But passion always belongs to the other, and thus emphasizes her lack.

Thus, it seems that Frau K. insists that she will make lack her passion, and that she will beat others with her stick. She must not shoot a broom. For if she shoots her stick, takes a shit, she will lose control. She will lose her essence, her passion, her self: *Ka-Ka*. The elementary phoneme, [*ka*], is all that remains of her being, the psychical representation of her imaginary instinct. She said: "*In meinen Traumen, er sprach meine Sprache*" ('In my dreams, he spoke my language'). But it is only a language of bodily sensations.

When Frau K. was threatened with non-being, what appeared foreclosed in the real were her symptoms. First is her delusion, that the Nazis wanted to control and take her mind; that is, to speak for her, render her speechless; and to kill her, the despised other, the Jew. Her passion to kill makes her a Nazi as well as the Jew who wants revenge. Whether she is victim or criminal it can only be resolved in the real, for she knows that they want to take her mind or kill her. Next are her hallucinations of smells and sounds, and of the signs on her body of disease. She smelled the gas that the Nazis used to kill the Jews. It was her gas, the olfactory image of her essence, which threatened to leave her and kill her. She hears the telephone ring and ring again to warn her that she must not lose control. And last, she has a phantom of that dirty, disgusting, unspeakable secret of syphilis inscribed on her body. That secret, her mother's secret now part of the family plot to which she can now belong alongside of those syphilitic ancestors, is her.

And now, the second phrase: "*wenn Gott schütze Rom*". The first word, *Gott*:

Gott=father	"Father had a new bathroom. I was forbidden to enter."
father=Cerberus	"His dog sat like Cerberus in front."
Cerberus=doctor	"I decided to be a doctor when they took my blood for the Wassermann, when they covered me with blood."
	"As a doctor, I do something more than talk."

The second word, *schütze* (the subjunctive):

schütze =protect, bar, shield (fence)	
schütze≠schiessen	
≠scheissen	"I was forbidden to enter."

The third word, *Rom*:

Rom=holy city	"The line of the divine is not for me."
Rom=room	"Six rooms parted me"
=bedroom/washroom	"Only my father could use that room."
	"The smell followed me for years."
=secret place	
=head (mind)	
=creativity	"When I was creative, I felt I had to keep it secret, or it would be taken away by grownups or doctors. I already was subconsciously against psychoanalysis."

Reconstructing the separate parts of these phrases yields the following:

"wenn Gott schütze Rom".

↓ ↓

father bedroom

↓ ↓

Cerberus bathroom

↓ ↓

doctor/I mind

protects

"if God shoots a broom".

father= stick

I= *Ka-Ka*

Only God the Father or Cerberus can protect her inner self, that self which is beginning to be anchored in language and recognizes the symbolic, with the acceptance of the name of the father. The father represents the law, which bars and alienates that secret place, the unconscious. The unconscious is also that place of creativity, which is a possibility for Frau K. except that something more fearful, something *verwerfen*, returns to haunt her like a ghost: emptiness.

5. Postscript

When I first treated Frau K., I wanted to help her repress her symptoms, and to reinstitute her self-esteem by helping her to return to work in medicine or art. Although she did get better, my desire to help, to want something for her that I thought best, impeded my understanding of her illness.

She repeatedly said: "My husband says I do nothing with my life. To be insane is proof enough that I made a lot out of my life. I'm alive in spite of it." To be alive and not be *wahnsinning* ('mad') like her father was her success, and helped to explain the (en)titling of paranoia querelans, with which she was introduced to me. At first I thought it was quaint, an echo of her husband's Viennese medical education, and Krapelin. Actually it was more of an echo from Frau K.'s personal past. About herself, she noted:

> I was a very egocentric, egotistic child; but not an egoistic one. I must have been lucky too, because I was more than once at the borderline of going insane, or commiting a crime of violence. Before I believed *only* in myself

> there was confusion. I wanted to be loved, but on the other hand I was frightened that someone might find the key to my personality. I would have been lost in love, and I knew in the end I would have been kicked again. I wanted to be loved, but I made it difficult; yes, impossible for those who never ever saw me.

Thus, the discourse of the other leads to chaos. The defense of offensiveness became not only a way of life, but a way to life. To her governess, Fräulein K., who asked her, What do you want? she replied: "I want, I want everything. More than all ... I want to show them."

Finally, there is this memory. Frau K. was telling me about her father's washroom, used only by him. She said:

> I asked him why? and he responded: *um etwas zu ziehen* ('Something to pull at', e.g., flush). He already had little to say. Papa was sick and dangerous. Hectar, his dog, had his place in front, like Cerberus. Never did I dare go in, but once in a while the door was open, and I could have a glimpse.

So, in the end, Frau K. had to be her own private place (a room with a hole) in which *ziehen* might occur. Frau K. said her father had little to say, but *ziehen*, rather than saying too little, says too much. When her father says nothing, there are too many meanings, an almost endless signification, which is the consequence of foreclosure and in which the psyche can only be represented through perception and sensation. Thus paradoxically *ziehen* can represent both presence and absence, whether one masturbates, defecates, or gives birth.

So, what more could I have done in treating Frau K.? Like Cerberus, I could help fence her out, away from the danger of an empty head, unspeakable. Yet in (at) the end, what was left was a hole in her head. The inside, the psyche, was once and for all externalized; and thus not empty but a presence, however diseased, there.

Notes

1. In a published interview with a hospitalized young man whom he called Gerard Primeau (in a play on a play on words, the name of the father foreclosed), Lacan detailed peculiarities of speech similar to that of Frau K. (Lacan 1980).
2. See Abraham (1987), wherein he describes how all body parts could signify illness – the illness, the passion of her blood – demonstrating desire as an endless metonymy.

References

Abraham, Nicolas

1987 "Notes on the phantom: a complement to Freud's metapsychology", (Translated by N. Rand.) *Critical Inquiry* 13, 287–292.

Freud, Sigmund

1900 *The interpretation of dreams.* S.E. IV &V. London: The Hogarth Press.

1905 *Three essays on the theory of sexuality.* S.E. VII, 125–243. London: The Hogarth Press.

1911 "Psycho-analytic notes on an autobiographical account of a case of paranoia (dementia paranoides)", S.E. XII, 3–82. London: The Hogarth Press.

1920 *Beyond the pleasure principle.* S.E. XVIII, 7–64. London: The Hogarth Press.

Lacan, Jacques

1966 Reponse à des étudiants en philosophie sur l'object de la psychanalyse, *Cahiers pour l'analyse* 3.

1977 *Écrits.* New York: W.W. Norton.

1980 "A Lacanian psychosis: interview by Jacques Lacan", in: Stuart Schneiderman (ed.), 19–41.

Leclaire, Serge

1958 "À la recherche des principles d'une psychotherapie des psychoses", *Évolution Psychiatrique* 2. Paris: Privat Didier.

Plato

1973 *Collected dialogues of Plato.* (Edited by Edith Hamilton & Huntington Cairns.). Princeton NJ: Princeton University Press.

Schneiderman, Stuart (ed.)

1980 *Returning to Freud: clinical psychoanalysis in the school of Lacan.* New Haven CT: Yale University Press.

List of contributors

Eugen Baer, Ph.D., is Professor of Philosophy at Hobart and William Smith Colleges in Geneva, New York.

Barnaby B. Barratt, Ph.D., is Adjunct Associate Professor in the Department of Psychiatry at Wayne State University and Professor of Clinical Psychology at the University of Detroit, Michigan.

Michael F. Basch, M.D., is a Training and Supervising Analyst at the Chicago Institute for Psychoanalysis and Professor of Psychiatry at Rush Medical College in Chicago, Illinois.

Phillip S. Epstein, M.D., is Assistant Professor of Psychiatry at Rush Medical College in Chicago, Illinois.

Arnold Goldberg, M.D., is a Training and Supervising Analyst at the Chicago Institute for Psychoanalysis and Professor of Psychiatry at Rush Medical College in Chicago, Illinois.

Matthias Kettner, Ph.D., is a Diplomate on the Faculty in Psychology at the Johann Wofgang Goethe Universitat in Frankfurt, West Germany.

Bonnie E. Litowitz, Ph.D., is the George and Mary Young Scholar and Adjunct Associate Professor in the Department of Psychiatry at Rush Medical College in Chicago, Illinois.

Bernard Rubin, M.D., is Professorial Lecturer in the Department of Psyschiatry at the University of Chicago in Chicago, Illinois.

Thure von Uexküll, M.D., is Professor Emeritus at the University of Ulm in Ulm, West Germany.

F. Eugene Yates, M.D., is the Ralph and Marjorie Crump Professor of Medical Engineering and Professor of Medicine in the Physiological Monitoring Unit at the University of California in Los Angeles, California.

Subject index

Bei Fragen zur Produktsicherheit wenden Sie sich bitte an:
If you have any questions regarding product safety,
please contact:

Walter de Gruyter GmbH
Genthiner Straße 13
10785 Berlin
productsafety@degruyterbrill.com